ACE Group Fitness Specialty Book

Aquatic Exercise

by Sabra Bonelli, M.S.

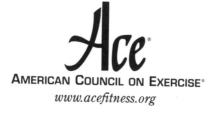

AMERICAN COUNCIL ON EXERCISE®
www.acefitness.org

Library of Congress Catalog Card Number: 00-111083

First edition
ISBN 1-890720-06-2
Copyright © 2001 American Council on Exercise (ACE)
Printed in the United States of America.

ABCDEF

Distributed by:
American Council on Exercise
P.O. Box 910449
San Diego, CA 92191-0449
(858) 535-8227
(858) 535-1778 (FAX)
www.acefitness.org

Managing Editor: Daniel Green
Design: Karen McGuire
Production: Ellen Goodwin
Manager of Publications: Christine J. Ekeroth
Assistant Editor: Jennifer Schiffer
Index: Bonny McLaughlin
Model: Jo-Anna Mitrano

Acknowledgments:
Thanks to the entire American Council on Exercise staff for their support and guidance through the process of creating this manual.

NOTICE
The fitness industry is ever-changing. As new research and clinical experience broaden our knowledge, changes in programming and standards are required. The authors and the publisher of this work have checked with sources believed to be reliable in their efforts to provide information that is complete and generally in accord with the standards accepted at the time of publication. However, in view of the possibility of human error or changes in industry standards, neither the authors nor the publisher nor any other party who has been involved in the preparation or publication of this work warrants that the information contained herein is in every respect accurate or complete, and they are not responsible for any errors or omissions or the results obtained from the use of such information. Readers are encouraged to confirm the information contained herein with other sources.

REVIEWERS

Angie Proctor is the executive director of the Aquatic Exercise Association and president of Personal Body Trainers, Inc. Specializing in both advanced land and water applications, Proctor brings creative and powerful programming to the world of fitness. Proctor is a leading international presenter, conducting programs on topics including aquatic fitness, personal training, management, and marketing.

Mary E. Sanders, M.S., is adjunct professor, Department of Health Ecology, University of Nevada, Reno; director of WaterFit/Wave Aerobics® & Golden Waves™; associate editor of ACSM's *Health & Fitness Journal* for the American College of Sports Medicine; editor/co-author of *YMCA Water Fitness for Health*; and developer of WaterFit and the Speedo® Aquatic Fitness System. Sanders conducts research in exercise physiology and educational leadership, trains instructors globally, and is an international presenter and author. She is the recipient of the 1997 IDEA, The Health & Fitness Association's Instructor of the Year award, the Aquatic Exercise Association's 2000 Global Award for Lifetime Achievement in Aquatic Fitness, and Fitness Educators of Older Adults Association's Fitness Educator of the Year, 2001. For more information on WaterFit/Wave Aerobics, and its more than 40 approved continuing education courses, contact ww.waterfit.com, www.dswfitness.com, or call 1-800-873-6759 for a course catalog.

TABLE OF
CONTENTS

INTRODUCTION

The American Council on Exercise (ACE) is pleased to include Aquatic Exercise as a Group Fitness Specialty Book. As the industry continues to expand, evolve, and redefine itself, it is only natural that aquatic exercise be recognized as a viable component of fitness. It has also become apparent that guidelines and criteria should be established so that this exercise modality can be practiced both safely and effectively. The intent of this book is to educate and give guidance to fitness professionals that wish to teach aquatic exercise. As with all areas of fitness, education is a continual process. ACE recognizes this is a broad subject requiring serious study and we encourage you to use the References and Suggested Reading to further your knowledge.

Chapter One

Introduction to Aquatic Exercise

Aquatic exercise is one of the most adaptable and versatile exercise training modalities. Water's natural resistance allows for a healthy, balanced workout with little risk of injury, while its buoyancy allows for minimal impact on joints. Because of water's myriad other properties, the aquatic environment truly provides a unique opportunity for participants to develop both physical and motor fitness, along with a variety of skills that aid movement on land. The versatility of water is reflected in the plethora of exercise options available to both participants and instructors, from arthritis and prenatal aquatics classes, to aquatics classes designed for training athletes. It is not surprising, then, that aquatic exercise participation is at an all-time high for both trained and untrained exercisers.

Growth

The earliest estimates of aquatic exercise participation approximated 200,000 in 1983 (Werner & Hoeger, 1995). By 1996, estimates of aquatic exercise participation in the United States had skyrocketed to more than 5 million, while most recent estimates have doubled that number to more than 10 million and growing (Aquatic Exercise Association, 1999). The 1999 IDEA Fitness Programs Survey of fitness business owners and program directors revealed the continued acceptance of aquatic exercise programming as a fitness staple, with 41% of respondents reporting they offer aquatic fitness programs (Ryan, 2000). A report by the Aquatic Exercise Association (1999) states that 85% of all public and private facility pools in the United States offer aquatic fitness programs.

Benefits

Aquatic exercise is unique in that it can provide training effects in all of the recommended fitness components (cardiorespiratory conditioning, muscular strength and endurance, and flexibility) with minimal risk of injury for exercisers of all ages and fitness levels. Because of water's versatility and safety, due mostly to its physical properties, it provides an ideal training medium for healthy fitness enthusiasts, competitive athletes, older adults, sedentary individuals, prenatal women, people recovering from injury or surgery, or those with chronic medical conditions such as arthritis or low-back pain.

One of the key benefits of water is injury prevention. Depending on water depth, the body is significantly less weightbearing in water than on land. Bearing less weight reduces joint stress and allows for full range of motion, while also allowing for greater overall intensity because of the water's resistance. Additionally, since buoyancy offsets the effects of gravity, participants can move unrestrained without fear of falling. Athletes can continue training in the cushioning environment of the water and maintain performance, while reducing the risk of injury from impact forces.

Another key benefit to aquatic exercise is progression. Properly using the properties of water (e.g., buoyancy, surface area, drag) allows exercisers to cater their workouts to their individual needs. Aquatic exercise involves progressive resistance by allowing for training in multiple ranges of motion and uninterrupted overload. Because of water's properties, an exerciser can instantly alter a movement, such as increasing or decreasing movement speed, to adjust intensity. Further, because movements in all directions are resisted, muscle conditioning can occur in a more time-efficient manner in water than on land. On land, movements are concentric when shortening a muscle against resistance, and gravity allows for eccentric muscle contraction when lengthening a muscle against resistance. In water, concentric conditioning for the prime muscle group occurs during the first half of the movement, just as on land (e.g., the hamstring muscle group during knee flexion). However, during the second half of the movement (knee extension in our example), the opposing muscle group (quadriceps) becomes the prime mover and also works concentrically. To target eccentric muscle contractions, aquatic equipment needs to be added, which also increases exercise intensity.

Aquatic exercise provides a large variety of additional benefits. It promotes postural stability and enhances balance, due to the effects of water currents on trunk musculature. Performing exercise in heart-to-neck level water strengthens respiratory musculature, due to the effects of hydrostatic pressure on the lungs. Water also provides a somewhat private, less-intimidating exercise environment for certain special populations, as being submerged allows them to feel comfortable while exercising, rather than feeling as though they are on display.

Considering these many benefits to exercising in the aquatic environment, most aquatic fitness experts agree that water training and land training should not be mutually exclusive, but rather used together to enhance the overall benefits of an exerciser's fitness program. Carol Kennedy, M.S., at Indiana University feels that "water should be regarded like any other resistance device.... Excluding water from a client's training program means you're leaving out an important piece of resistance 'equipment'" (Sanders, 1999, 1).

Water Research

During the past decade, numerous research studies have shown without question the value and versatility of aquatic fitness as an exercise modality. Its widespread and growing popularity among exercisers of all levels, ages, and abilities simply validates these research outcomes.

Cardiorespiratory Fitness

To achieve cardiorespiratory benefits from any exercise modality, the American College of Sports Medicine (ACSM) training guidelines state that exercise must be conducted within a specified intensity range, usually measured in oxygen consumption, or $\dot{V}O_2$ (ACSM, 1998). Early research on acute bouts of water fitness showed that participants can reach and sustain work in this required intensity range during a water fitness class (Cassady & Nielsen, 1992). Later studies showed that consistent participation in repeated bouts of aquatic exercise can significantly improve cardiorespiratory fitness (Hoeger et al., 1993; Ruoti, Troup, & Berger, 1994; Sanders & Rippee, 1993). However, while the relationship between oxygen consumption and heart rate is highly predictable on land, this is not the case in water. For complete information on monitoring intensity and the heart-rate response to aquatic exercise, see Chapter 5.

Muscular Conditioning and Flexibility

With the dynamic properties of water, it is no surprise that research has found aquatic exercise improves both muscle strength and muscle endurance. Examining the effects of rhythmic exercise, movements in both shallow and deep water elicit muscle strength and endurance gains (Sanders & Rippee, 1993). Studies that examined only shallow water rhythmic exercise yielded the same results (Hoeger et al., 1993; Ruoti, Troup, & Berger, 1994). And still other studies looking at the effects of rhythmic exercise in deep water alone demonstrated that both muscle strength and endurance gains are possible (Baretta, 1993).

In the studies conducted by Baretta (1993) and Hoeger et al. (1993), aquatic exercise improved flexibility in muscle groups. It stands to reason that performing stretches in water should provide similar flexibility gains as experienced when those stretches are performed on land. Unfortunately, research to date has not provided conclusive evidence of the flexibility benefits of aquatic exercise (YMCA of the USA, 2000). However, research does confirm the ability of aquatic exercise to enhance active range of motion in diseased and older individuals (see Therapeutic and Functional Training, page 7).

Weight Management

Many exercisers place considerable emphasis on weight management when selecting and adhering to a fitness routine. For this reason, the extent to which aquatic exercise affects weight control is of great importance. Due to some faulty, preliminary research that found it to be ineffective for weight or fat loss (Gwinup, 1987), there has been ample controversy in this area of aquatic exercise research. Two significant studies found that regular participation in aquatic exercise classes does in fact promote body-fat loss (Abraham, Szczerba, & Jackson, 1994; Hoeger et al., 1993). Unfortunately, two other studies yielded the conflicting results that aquatic exercise does not reduce body-fat levels in adults (Campbell et al., 1990; Ruoti, Troup, & Berger, 1994). However, another more recent study again found aquatic exercise effective in reducing body fat (Sanders, Constantino, & Rippee, 1997). Because of research difficulties when dealing with both exercise and diet, which are inextricably related, the current answer to the weight management and aquatic exercise question is a definite "maybe." However, as Evans (1996) states, "A number of research studies have indicated that rhythmic, upright exercise in the water can increase energy expenditure…[and] the additional energy output *should* lead to the control of weight and body fat." Future research in this area will eventually clarify the matter.

Bone Loss

A 1994 study in Japan by Tsukahara et al. investigated bone loss in healthy postmenopausal women who participated in aquatic exercise programs. Comparing women who had been aquatic exercise participants for an average of approximately three years with beginners new to water fitness (and to sedentary controls) revealed significantly greater bone density in the long-time aquatic exercisers. Additional longitudinal results revealed significantly increased bone mineral density in the aquatic exercise participants (both beginners and long-time regulars), versus a decrease each year seen in the sedentary controls. The researchers concluded consistent aquatic exercise participation may be an important bone loss prevention method.

A more recent study by Bravo et al. (1997) looked at the effects of a weightbearing aquatic exercise program on postmenopausal women with low bone mineral mass. Participants exercised three times per week for 60 minutes per session in waist-level water for 12 months. In comparing pre- and post-test results, flexibility, agility, muscle strength and endurance, and cardiorespiratory endurance increased significantly. However, bone mineral density of the femoral neck (commonly fractured portion of the hip) did not change, while spinal bone mineral density actually decreased significantly during the year. The study's authors concluded that although the aquatic exercise program used in the study was shown to improve functional fitness, additional research is needed to identify specific exercises that can safely promote a positive bone response.

Therapeutic and Functional Training

The benefits of water therapy for rehabilitation have long been known (Koury, 1996). The properties of water, such as buoyancy, help prevent injuries because of reduced impact (Sanders, 2000). Further, hydrostatic pressure reduces tissue swelling and blood pooling in the extremities during exercise, and increases metabolic waste product excretion (Becker & Cole, 1997).

Functional training in water has also been shown to improve performance of activities of daily living (ADLs) for a variety of populations. Sufferers of chronic back pain who undergo therapeutic aquatic exercise programs experience reduced pain and improved ADL performance (Landgridge & Phillips, 1988; Smit & Harrison, 1991). Studies that looked at joint motion and ADL performance for persons with arthritis and rheumatic diseases also reported decreased pain and increased range of motion after water therapy exercise programs (Suomi & Lindaur, 1997; Templeton, Booth, & Kelly, 1996).

Results have been just as positive in healthy (non-diseased or injured) older adults who gained functional postural mobility through aquatic exercise (Simmons & Hansen, 1996). An aquatic exercise study conducted through the Sanford Center on Aging at the University of Nevada, Reno evaluated ADL performance in older adults (Sanders, Constantino, & Rippee, 1997). The authors found that water training significantly improved functional abilities, increased muscle strength and flexibility, decreased body fat, and improved self-esteem.

Athletic Training

Although still thought of by many as an exercise mode for the elderly or less fit, research repeatedly demonstrates the efficacy of aquatic exercise training for athletes. Two studies looked at the effects of deep-water running and athletic performance. Wilber and colleagues (1996) concluded that deep-water running may serve effectively as an alternative training program to land running in trained endurance athletes. They found that aerobic performance after a six-week deep-water running program yielded comparable results in the water-trained and land-trained groups. A later study by Bushman et al. (1997) also concluded that deep-water runners can maintain on-land running performance after replacing land training with a four-week deep-water running program.

A third study on athletic performance (Stemm, 1993) examined the effects of plyometric training in water versus on land. Both water- and land-trained groups had similar increases in vertical jump measures after training in knee-deep water. Other studies in four-feet-deep and chest-deep water yielded similar results (Kolovou & Eksten, 1998), continuing to demonstrate the effectiveness of water training for athletes.

Chapter Two

Exercise Science In Water

T he knowledge and skills required to lead safe and effective land-based group fitness classes is extensive. Teaching in the water environment requires many of the same skills, including the ability to work with groups and the knowledge of exercise science and physiological principles. Additionally, aquatic fitness instructors must have a thorough understanding of water's physical properties and how to best apply those properties to movement design. Knowledge of the physical laws of the water environment allows the instructor to lead participants in exercises that provide maximum benefit. The key scientific principles that affect movement in water include buoyancy and drag forces. The key properties of water that act on the body include action/reaction, resistance, inertia, hydrostatic pressure, speed and force, and surface area and leverage.

Buoyancy

Archimedes' principle states that, "When a body at rest is partially or totally immersed in any fluid, it experiences an upward thrust equal to the weight of the fluid displaced" (Kolovou & Eksten, 1998). This principle describes the buoyant property of water. Stated another way, buoyancy is the upward lift or force that water exerts on the body when partially or completely submerged. The magnitude of the buoyant force exerted on the body is dependent on the weight of water displaced, which varies depending on the weight, size, density, body fat, and lung capacity of the submerged body.

A 150-pound aquatic exercise participant with a low body-fat percentage who is lean and muscular has a more dense, compact body and will displace a relatively small amount of water. If the participant's body weighs more than the amount of water displaced, the participant will sink. In this example, the amount of buoyancy force pressing up against the body equals a small amount, because only a small amount of water is displaced. Another 150-pound aquatic exercise participant with a high body-fat percentage and a smaller amount of muscle mass will displace a larger amount of water. Because fat is less dense than water, the amount of water displaced will be greater than the weight of the body and the participant will float. In this case, because of the large amount of water displaced, a large amount of buoyancy force is generated.

Due to the upward lift of buoyancy, a body is less weight-bearing in water. The effects of gravity are reduced and joint compression minimized, which reduces the potential for injury. The degree to which these benefits of buoyancy take effect depends on how far the body is immersed in water. Although the percentages vary based on gender and body composition, in general a body submerged to the waist bears 50% of its weight. Submersion to the chest bears 25% to 35%, while submersion to the neck bears only 10% of the body weight (Aquatic Exercise Association, 2000). Considering these numbers, it is easy to see the appeal of aquatic exercise for people who cannot exercise under the full weightbearing conditions of land, such as older adults needing reduced joint and connective tissue stress.

It is also easy to understand the need to adjust both balance and coordination when exercising in the water. On land, a person's center of gravity is typically located in the hip area. When submerged in water the body doesn't rotate around its center of gravity as it does on land, but rather around its center of buoyancy. The center of buoyancy is the lightest part of the body for its size, which is typically in the chest area where the lungs are located. The lungs are light for their size when filled with air, and are the most buoyant part of the body (YMCA of the USA, 1999).

When designing movements for an aquatic exercise class, the centers of gravity and buoyancy should be vertically aligned so the body is relatively stable. When moved out of vertical alignment, participants are at increased risk of musculoskeletal injury. Therefore, care must be taken when designing traveling moves and transitions. The principle of buoyancy itself can be usefully applied to movement design. Buoyancy can assist or resist movements in water, much like the effects of gravity on land. Movements toward the pool surface are called buoyancy "assisted," as buoyancy acts to provide additional vertical lift, which assists the movement. On the other hand, the term buoyancy "resisted" describes moves of a buoyant object toward the bottom of the pool. Floating movements on the water surface are referred to as buoyancy "supported" (Aquatic Exercise Association, 2000). Table 2.1 shows a comparison of gravity assisted/resisted muscle work on land and buoyancy-assisted/resisted muscle work in water.

Table 2.1
Comparison of Muscle Land Work (Standing Upright) vs. Water Exercise

Land Exercise	
Assisted	**Resisted**
Triceps	Biceps
Abdominals	Erector spinae
Adductors	Abductors
Latissimus dorsi	Deltoids
Water Exercise	
Assisted	**Resisted**
Abductors	Adductors
Deltoids	Latissimus dorsi
Biceps	Triceps

Adapted from Kennedy & Sanders, 1995. Reproduced with permission of IDEA, The Health & Fitness Association, (800) 999-IDEA or (858) 535-8979: www.ideafit.com.

Drag Forces

According to the *Aquatic Fitness Professional Manual* (Aquatic Exercise Association, 2000), "Drag is the most significant force available in the aquatic environment." In the water, drag is the force that opposes motion. Drag can occur in any direction based on the movement performed, whereas buoyancy occurs only in the vertical direction. Because of this, an experienced aquatic fitness instructor can manipulate drag forces to provide a variety of intensity options for any movement. Doing this allows class participants to select the movement intensity that most appropriately challenges them based on their individual fitness level.

Drag force is directly related to the amount of surface area and smoothness of a moving object. For example, when moving the hand through water, a cupped hand will encounter more drag force than a flat hand. If moving a piece of water-resistance equipment such as an aquatic dumbbell, drag force will be greater as the frontal surface area of the dumbbell increases (a square-ended versus circular-ended dumbbell). Streamlining the moving object will decrease drag force and decrease movement intensity. For example, a slicing hand will encounter less drag force than a flat hand. Drag forces are also affected by velocity (the speed/direction of movement) and the overall shape of the object.

Action and Reaction

Newton's Third Law of Motion tells us that for every action there is an equal and opposite reaction. Although not always apparent on land, the uniqueness of the water environment causes the paired forces of action and reaction to become obvious. For instance, the action of applying force to push the body down in water causes a reaction of the body being pushed up. Similarly, kicking a leg forward produces a reactive force that presses the body backward. The more force applied in an action, the greater the reactive force generated.

Just as buoyancy can be used to alter intensity by assisting or resisting movement, the action/reaction principle can also be used to adjust intensity when designing water fitness movements. For example, the action of pushing the arms forward generates a reactive force that pushes or travels the body backward. Intensity can be increased by simultaneously performing a movement that resists travel backward, such as kicking backward (which pushes the body forward). The intensity increases because the reactive forces created by the arms oppose those of the legs, causing greater water turbulence and increased resistance. Intensity can be decreased, then, by using reactive forces that assist other reactive forces (e.g., pushing the arms forward and kicking forward).

Resistance

Viscosity is the friction that occurs between water molecules that causes them to adhere to each other (cohesion) and to a submerged body (adhesion). It is this viscous and dense nature of water that provides constant multi-dimensional resistance to movement. When the body's weight is supported by water, the friction between water molecules causes resistance to motion, which requires the muscles to work harder than if they were moving through air. In fact, movement under water creates on the average approximately 12 to 15 times more resistance than movement on land (Curry, 1997; Sanders, 2000).

Water resistance can be altered in numerous ways. Turbulent (irregular) water flow creates currents to work against, which enhance resistance, whereas streamlined water flow minimizes resistance (think of an efficient lap swimmer). Faster movement also creates greater resistance, as does increasing the surface area of a moving object or the lever length of a moving limb. The unique and instantly variable resistance of water encourages agonist/antagonist muscle balance and enhances the development of both muscle strength and muscle endurance. The more work required of the muscle to push, press, or pull in the water, the more intense the workout.

Inertia

Newton's First Law of Motion, the Law of Inertia, describes the tendency of a body to remain in a state of constant motion, uniform motion, or rest, until acted upon by an outside force. In air, inertia causes the need for muscular effort to move a limb. In water, inertia must also be overcome to start, stop, or change the direction of movement. For example, effort is required to overcome inertia and begin walking forward. Once moving, inertia must again be overcome to change direction or stop walking. In water, unlike air, walking forward creates currents that resist any change in movement. The viscous properties of water, which provide even more resistance to movement, cause the effects of inertia to be greater in water than on land.

Inertia can be used to either increase or decrease exercise intensity in water. Directional changes that create opposing water currents to move against increase exercise intensity. Increases can also be instigated by quickly repeating moves back and forth or continually starting/stopping movement sequences. Movements used to increase intensity can greatly challenge participants' balance, stability, body control, and posture. Therefore, it is critical to also instruct participants on the use of inertia to decrease intensity (e.g., avoiding moving forward) to ensure an individualized workout.

Hydrostatic Pressure

Compression, or the pressure exerted by molecules of water on an immersed body, is referred to as hydrostatic pressure. This pressure is exerted equally against all surfaces (the weight of the water presses against all sides of a submerged body), and increases as the depth and density of water increase. Although hydrostatic pressure does not directly affect water exercise intensity, it is an important physical law to understand because of its influence on the vascular and respiratory systems. Hydrostatic pressure acts as a "bandage" to compress capillaries to assist the return of venous blood to the heart and to decrease swelling in the extremities, especially the feet, where pressure and water depth are greatest (Forster, 1997). Further, hydrostatic pressure on the chest cavity can cause labored breathing when the lungs are submerged. While this pressure can be useful in conditioning the respiratory muscles, it may be problematic for people with respiratory disorders (Aquatic Exercise Association, 2000). Participants with hypertension should be encouraged to gradually increase water depth, as hydrostatic pressure may cause an initial rise in systolic blood pressure upon immersion (YMCA of the USA, 2000).

Speed, Force, and Acceleration

Speed describes the rate at which a movement or activity can be performed, while *force* is what is applied to an object to cause its acceleration or deceleration. Force alters movement speed. For land exercise, speed depends on how fast the limbs move, irrespective of air resistance. Speed in water is different than on land, because of certain properties of water described in this chapter. While assuming a vertical body position in water, faster movements create greater intensity. Moving faster also results in greater drag and resistance, which in turn requires more muscular work/force for movement (YMCA of the USA, 2000).

Acceleration describes change of motion, or how fast a change in direction or speed will occur when a force is applied. Greater force causes greater acceleration, which in turn causes greater speed of movement. Acceleration can alter water exercise intensity (for instance, when participants use their limbs to push against the water's resistance or to push against the pool bottom with more force). Other water properties, namely buoyancy and inertia, can also affect participants' ability to accelerate a movement and thereby increase the resistance and intensity of exercise.

For all participants, movement range of motion must not be compromised when trying to increase movement speed, force, or intensity. It is critically important that water exercisers perform movements with control at all times, rather than simply equating faster movements with more intense exercise. Communicate to participants that it is never acceptable to increase movement speed at the expense of proper form during movement execution.

Surface Area and Leverage

Surface area and leverage are variables used in aquatic exercise to increase movement intensity. The size and shape of an object's surface area affects intensity by altering the drag force and resistance generated by movement. An "object" may be the entire body, a limb (arm or leg), or a piece of equipment. Surface area also impacts the movement speed capable of being reached, without jeopardizing range of motion.

Leverage also relates to surface area. Movements using longer levers (limbs) increase the surface area of the body part being moved. Again, greater surface area creates greater drag force, resistance, and ultimately, an increase in the overall intensity of the movement. An example of changing lever length to increase required work would be substituting a knee lift (a shortened lever) with a straight leg kick (a move with a longer limb that encounters greater resistance and requires more force/work to perform).

Chapter Three

Working Positions and Basic Aquatic Moves

A s with every other exercise modality, aquatic exercise has certain staple movements about which all instructors must be knowledgeable. These basic moves and skills are the foundation of safe and effective aquatic exercise. Stabilization skills should be taught to beginning aquatic exercise participants before the start of their first class, and should be reviewed frequently with all levels of participants to ensure their competence and comfort in performing them. Instructors also need to clearly understand the different working positions available in aquatic exercise, as well as basic water moves, to appropriately design an aquatic fitness class.

Basic Stabilization Skills

Recovery to Standing

Although some aquatic exercise class participants may be superior swimmers, most will not have a swimming background and thus will not be confident in their water skills. The extent of these exercisers' participation in class will be affected by fear of the water. For instance, falling face down or up to a horizontal position can be extremely scary, and can potentially hyperextend the back (YMCA of the USA, 2000). Because of the possibility of losing footing and/or balance during movements, it is important to teach participants the skill of recovery to a stand. In deep water, the essential skill is recovery to a vertical position rather than to "standing" (which is not possible in deep water); however, it is taught the same way.

In teaching recovery to a stand, first explain to participants that regaining a vertical orientation should be done from the supine position to protect the back. Have students begin face down and horizontal in the water. Teach them to turn their head to one side, and as the body follows the head, continue rolling over to the supine, face-up horizontal position. From here, "recovery" is performed. Participants should relax the body and pull the knees into the chest. Next, participants should scoop under the knees with the arms to shift the body forward (vertical), lift their chin, and stand up (Sanders & Rippee, 1993).

Sculling

Sculling is one of the fundamental skills aquatic exercisers can use for balance, lift, and assistance with traveling or direction changes. It is essentially a figure-8 motion with the palms down, and involves use of the hands, wrists, and arms to help stabilize the body in neutral posture. Due to the principles of action/reaction and buoyancy, when the large flat surface of the hand pushes down against the water while sculling, the body is lifted upward. In this way sculling provides lift, assists in proper posture, and helps participants to balance. Sculling motions can also aid exercisers in traveling or resisting travel with large figure-8 movements, which can produce propulsion and add to the exercise intensity experienced by the upper body. Debbie Miles-Dutton (1996) describes how to teach sculling to beginning water exercisers.

> "To teach beginners this skill, have them close their eyes and imagine sitting in a warm pile of sand. Have them open their arms away from their sides, palms down, and begin to move their hands back and forth as though they were smoothing the sand. Have them begin with small, light, figure-8 movements; move on to larger, sweeping motions; and then do the motions quickly."

Proper Body Alignment

To ensure the safety and effectiveness of any water movement, it is critical that participants maintain proper body alignment at all times. Most movements in aquatic exercise classes originate from the *ready position*, also known as the *athletic stance* (YMCA of the USA, 2000). This position involves standing tall with the chest out, shoulders retracted and depressed, chin neutral, abdominals contracted with a neutral spine, and the body centered (aligned ears, shoulders, hips, and heels). Closely monitor participants' body position throughout each class, and regularly correct and modify movement in participants having trouble maintaining correct posture.

Working Positions

Extended Position

In the extended working position, participants stand tall and maintain normal posture with proper body alignment, as described in the previous section. In this position, sometimes called the "anchored" position, one leg continually touches the pool bottom. Movements are performed with the body extended upright, which largely involves the core muscles and reduces impact forces (similar to low-impact aerobics in traditional group fitness programming). Moves initiated from the extended position might include knee lifts, kicks, and water walking.

Rebound Position

In the rebound position, participants forcefully press against the pool bottom to move up vertically. The greater force participants apply to the upward push, the greater their movement is accelerated and the more their movement is affected by drag, resistance, and gravity. Impact and intensity also increase with rebounding, as the movement requires greater speed and power to be successfully accomplished. The rebound position can be used in moves such as jumping, rocking, and extended-position moves where more intensity is desired.

Neutral Position

To perform aquatic exercise movements from the neutral position, exercisers lower their bodies into the water to heart- or neck-level, keeping their feet on the pool bottom. Their feet may tap or slide softly along the pool bottom, while their arms move through the water both vertically and horizontally, at or below the surface of the water. Key to the effectiveness of this working position is maintaining proper alignment of the trunk and a neutral spine. This may pose a challenge for some participants, as full submersion of the body causes an increase in both buoyancy and hydrostatic pressure. The benefit to the neutral position, though, involves proper use of the heightened effect of buoyancy. According to Sanders and Curry (YMCA of the USA, 2000), "…with the assistance of buoyancy, long lever horizontal moves are more effective. As more of the lever is submerged in a resistive environment, intensity can be increased through leverage, [form] drag, action/reaction, and speed."

Suspended Position

The suspended position is the greatest way to eliminate impact in aquatic exercise. In this position, participants lift their feet off the pool bottom and their bodies are held up completely by the water's buoyancy. Participants work their arms and legs without touching the ground, as they would in deep water exercise (the entire class is conducted in the suspended position). Although impact is minimized, the properties of water (i.e., inertia, resistance, and leverage) become even greater factors in moving. Additionally, because of greater buoyancy and minimized gravity, balance becomes difficult. This position requires great skill and practice for full effectiveness and safety.

Basic Aquatic Moves

Basic Cardiovascular Aquatic Moves

When designing exercises for cardiovascular conditioning in shallow or transitional water depth, there are six basic moves: walking, jogging, kicking, rocking, jumping, and scissors (Sanders & Rippee, 1993). For all six of these base moves, you can progress the intensity, difficulty, and complexity, and create movement variation by using the different water properties to your advantage, as described in Chapter 2.

Walking

Walking in water involves traveling the body through water just like walking on land. It involves striding in waist- to chest-deep water with neutral spinal alignment and vertical posture (avoiding a forward lean). Variations include walking backward or sideways, walking with toes pointed out, walking with high knees, and walking on the heels or toes. These variations help provide muscle balance by altering the muscles used. Additional variety (and intensity) can be accomplished by using the arms out of water, or in water to stroke forward or backward, or to punch or scull while walking. Beginners should focus on leg movements first, progressing to add arm movements only when capable of maintaining balance and form.

Jogging

Jogging in place (a thermal move often used to keep body temperature up in cooler water) involves hopping in place from one foot to the other, keeping a flexed knee on the other leg at the ending position. Jogging with a travel is essentially walking while rebounding, adding both intensity and impact to the movement. Erect posture is critical to properly perform the jog. Variations to the jog include running and mambos.

To add intensity, the arm variations as described in the walking section can be used with the same precautions for progressing participants.

Kicking

To perform a kick, participants lift one leg while the other remains stationary (standing, bouncing, or suspended if applicable). As with all moves, proper kicking requires upright posture with a lifted ribcage and neutral spine. When kicking, observe that participants do not hyperextend the knee or curl the torso or pelvis in the direction of the kick, which may be toward the front, side, or back. Variations of the kick include fan kicks, Russian kicks (alternating kicks so the second leg kicks while the first leg returns from kicking), knee lifts, and hamstring curls. A deep-water or suspended variation is flutter kicks, which are quick alternating lower-leg extension movements that often require buoyancy equipment and are performed from the seated or supine position. With kicks, participants should first focus on arm movements that aid balance by working them in opposition to the legs, and then progress to arm moves that increase resistance, action/reaction, and leverage.

Rocking

Rocking involves shifting the weight from one leg to the other, usually with a rebounding or bouncing motion. The most common rocking movements are the rocking horse and the pendulum. In the rocking-horse move, one leg lifts forward while standing or bouncing on the other. As the lifted leg returns to the pool floor, the other leg lifts backward. A variation on this move is to alter the lever length of the leg, performing the rocking horse with flexed versus straightened legs. The pendulum is a rocking move where the legs are alternately lifted out to the sides. To increase the intensity of rocking movements, participants could include arm movements to create turbulence or currents in the water (action/reaction principle), which challenge balance and stability.

Jumping

A jump is a rebound landing on one or both feet. Jumps in the rebound position are very high-intensity movements that increase impact, while jumps in the neutral position can moderately increase intensity without much additional impact. Safe jumping is important, so emphasize landing toe-ball-heel with soft knees (lengthened but not locked) directly over the ankles. To increase the intensity of jumps, participants can begin and end in deeper knee flexion, which increases the distance traveled under water, or they can change the water depth at which the jumps are performed. Variations to the basic jump that increase intensity include jumping jacks, traveling jumps, jumping with a twist, frog-leg jumps, and leaps.

Scissors

The scissor move can best be described as moving the arms and legs simultaneously in a cross-country skiing motion. As with the other five basic moves and their variations, intensity can be progressed by making larger movements versus smaller, rebounding or working from a suspended position versus the neutral position, or traveling the move versus performing it in place.

Basic Muscle-Conditioning Aquatic Moves

The basic water moves for muscular strength and endurance training are similar to muscle strengthening land movements, and they must be performed with proper body alignment. Common exercises include elbow flexion/extension, shoulder flexion/extension, horizontal shoulder abduction/adduction, deltoid lateral raises, knee flexion/extension, squats, lunges, and abdominal curls. To obtain the added benefits of strength training during water movements, adequate resistance must be applied to the working muscles. Resistance can be added from a stationary position by varying the movement range of motion and increasing movement tempo or speed. Adding traveling to utilize the properties of water can also make exercises more difficult (e.g., walking forward while performing a bicep curl). Using equipment is the other common way to ensure the effectiveness of muscle strength and endurance exercises (e.g., using buoyancy equipment such as dumbbells for shoulder adduction, or webbed gloves to increase surface area when performing tricep extensions). The following photos demonstrate some of the previously listed conditioning exercises, some of which utilize water equipment (Figures 1–6).

Figure 1
Bicep curl walking forward; Walking forward as the bicep curl is performed forces the bicep muscle to overcome the additional resistance created by moving water versus still water.
a. Starting position
b. Ending position

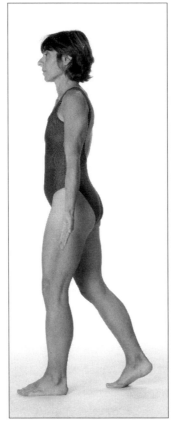

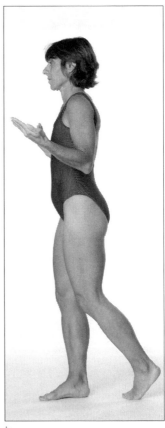

a.

b.

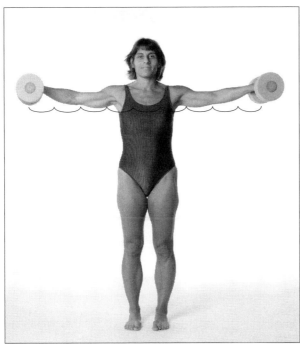

Figure 2
Shoulder adduction with dumbbells; Buoyancy dumbbells add resistance by requiring the shoulders to push the dumbbells down with greater force.
a. Starting position
b. Ending position

a.

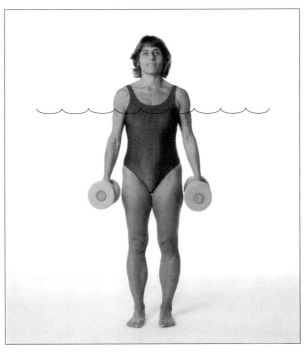

b.

Figure 3
Tricep Extension
with webbed
gloves;
Webbed gloves
add resistance
to the tricep
extension by in-
creasing the
surface area of
the palm-open
hand as it
moves through
water.
a. Starting
    position
b. Ending
    position

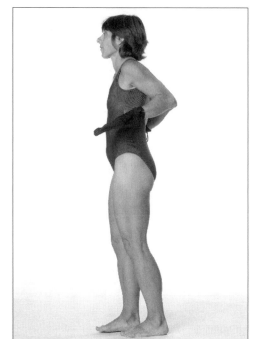

a.

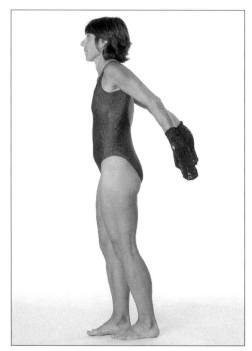

b.

Figure 4
Squat with kickboard;
For added resistance during the squat, a kickboard can be held in the arms parallel to the water level, adding to the downward force that must be exerted to perform the squat in water.

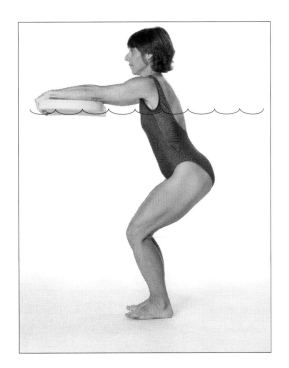

Figure 5
Lunge

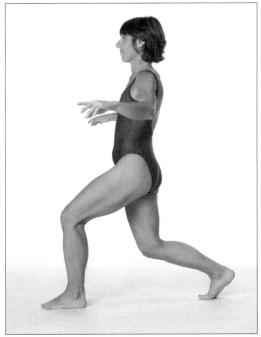

Figure 6

Crunches;
Abdominal
stabilization
with hip flexion
using the noodle;
Abdominal
exercises can
be performed
using a noodle
to hold the body
suspended
in water.
a. Starting position
b. Ending position

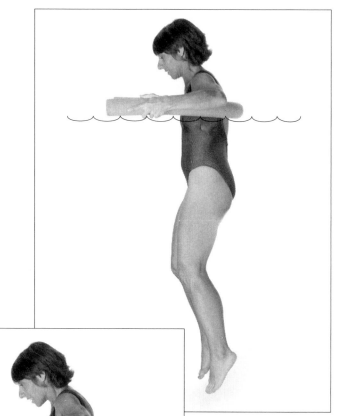

a.

b.

Basic Aquatic Stretches

Stretches for flexibility conditioning as part of an aquatic exercise class are essentially the same stretches performed in a land group exercise class. Based on the types of movements executed in class, stretches should be done for the quadriceps, hamstrings, hip flexors, gastrocnemius, abductors, adductors, back, chest, shoulders, arms, and neck. Stretches will differ depending on temperature. If the water is warmer, stretches may be relaxation-oriented. If the water is colder, stretches might need to be held static at the stretching muscle group, while the rest of the body continues to move (e.g., jogging while performing shoulder stretches). Sample stretches are presented here through photos and brief descriptions (Figures 7–15).

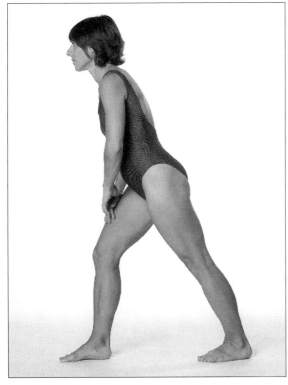

Figure 7
A gastrocnemius (calf) stretch

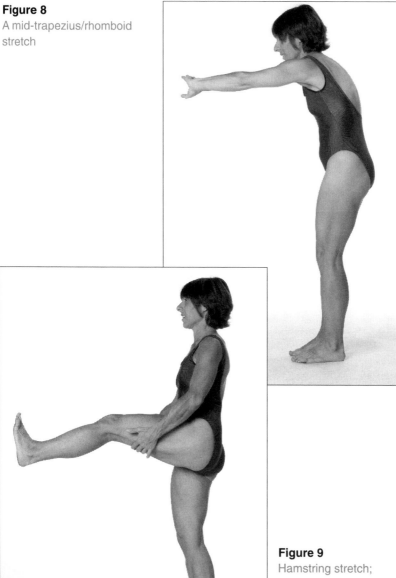

Figure 8
A mid-trapezius/rhomboid
stretch

Figure 9
Hamstring stretch;
An effective stretch of
the hamstring can be
performed in water by
holding the leg in an
extended position.

Figure 10
Adductor stretch;
Using the resistance of the
water, an adductor stretch
can be performed by sliding
laterally to "drag" the
stretching leg.

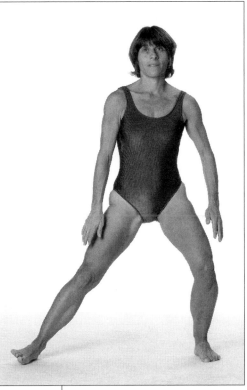

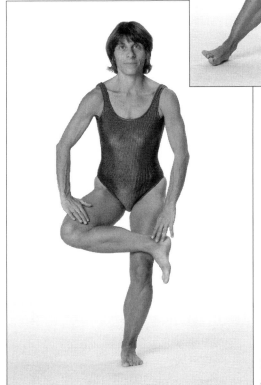

Figure 11
An abductor stretch

Figure 12
A hip flexor stretch

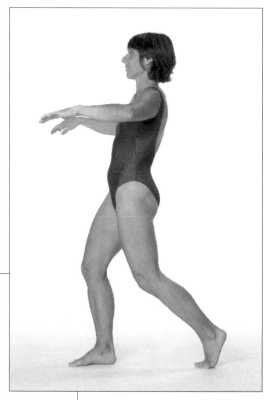

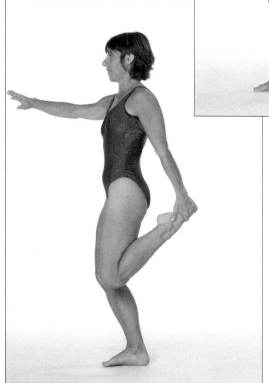

Figure 13
A quadricep stretch

Figure 14
Pectoral stretch;
Using the resistance of the
water, an effective pectoral
muscle stretch can be
performed by extending the
arms backwards while walking
forward.

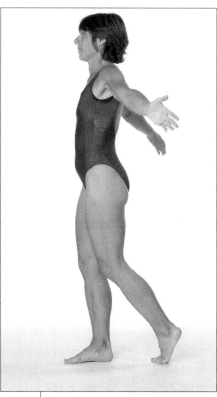

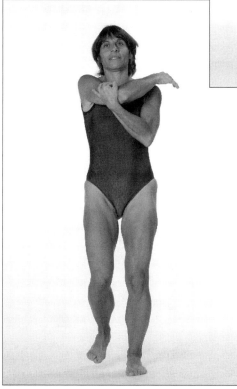

Figure 15
Deltoid stretch;
To avoid excessive
chilling, the deltoid
stretch can be
performed while jogging.

Chapter Four

Aquatic Exercise Equipment

The main purpose of most aquatic exercise equipment is to increase intensity, as without equipment there are fewer movement modifications, which limits the possibility of progression in fitness gains. Do not underestimate the value of professional aquatic exercise equipment, as it can play a vital role in keeping participants both interested and properly challenged. Today, a wide array of aquatic equipment can aid participants of all ages and fitness levels in efficiently achieving their workout goals. This selection of equipment includes items that are either held by aquatic exercise participants or are attached to their bodies. Equipment can be used to enhance buoyancy and/or to create additional overload for resistance training. More specifically, different pieces of aquatic equipment provide balance, resistance, traction, safety, comfort, warmth, buoyancy, drag, cardiovascular work, sports training, and functional exercises. You need to clearly understand the purpose and proper use of the different types of equipment, so you can educate participants on the needed safety skills. Further, understanding the equipment options and their applications will help ensure that you are selecting equipment that is appropriate for the needs and abilities of each class.

Choosing the Right Equipment

Most aquatic fitness instructors will have to decide which types of equipment can provide the most benefit to all populations, and which can be used for multiple applications. Most often, funding is the determining factor in aquatic equipment purchases, as there are often limited finances available. Usually instructors have little say in determining which pieces of aquatic equipment are purchased, and must instead work with what is made available to them. Your responsibility then, is to determine the appropriateness of the available equipment for your class populations.

One of the first things to consider when determining equipment use is participant make-up. What are the characteristics of the majority of the participants in class? Are they primarily seniors or younger athletes? Are they beginners or advanced water exercisers? Do class participants have a wide range of skills and abilities, which makes your job even more challenging? Keeping the participant profile in mind, the next step is to objectively think through a variety of considerations to determine the appropriateness of a piece of aquatic equipment. Experts recommend using an established set of criteria to evaluate aquatic fitness equipment, such as that presented in Table 4.1. For all equipment, first consider its primary purpose (cardiovascular fitness, muscle strength or endurance, flexibility, or weight management). Next, determine which muscles are involved in movements, which water properties are involved, to whom the equipment is best suited, and the skills needed for proper use. Answering these questions can ensure appropriate exercise design for any piece of aquatic equipment, so exercisers achieve their goals in the safest manner.

Table 4.1
Evaluation Criteria for Selecting Aquatic Equipment

---

1. What is (are) the equipment's purpose(s) and objective(s) for water exercise?

2. What exercises can be performed with the equipment? Are they functional and effective?

3. Which water properties are used?

4. Can the equipment be used through various exercise progressions, making it suitable for participants of all ages and fitness levels?

5. What are the potential risks?

6. What skills are needed to use the equipment?

7. How much does the equipment cost, and what is its expected longevity?

8. Is the equipment easily stored, replaced, and transported?

Twynham,1998. Reproduced with permission of IDEA, The Health & Fitness Association, (800) 999-IDEA or (858) 535-8979: www.ideafit.com. Adapted from Sanders & Rippee, 1993 & Sanders, 1999, 3, with permission from WaterFit/Wave Aerobics: www.waterfit.com.

The two main types of aquatic equipment for use in the class setting include equipment that is *water-specific* (buoyancy and surface area equipment) and equipment that is used for *land/water integration* (YMCA of the USA, 2000). It is beyond the scope of this book to review the proper use of all types of aquatic equipment. Therefore, the sections that follow will review the basic purpose of the different equipment categories, provide a list of specific pieces that fall within that category, and review a few examples of how a particular piece of equipment can be used.

Buoyancy Equipment

B uoyancy equipment floats in water and can provide buoyant support to the entire body or to particular limbs. The purpose of this type of equipment is to create additional upward thrust or lift to generate overload. With greater lift (buoyancy force) pressing the body or limbs up, downward movements require increased resistance. The actual amount of overload created through greater resistance is highly variable, based on individual body composition, water depth, and the type of equipment used. The density and volume/size of a product greatly affect the amount of buoyancy and resistance it can provide (larger pieces of equipment provide greater buoyancy and require greater force/resistance).

Buoyancy equipment is usually made of foam, although some types are air-inflated. Whole-body buoyancy devices are used to place participants in the suspended position, in which the body is held up in the water with the feet off the pool bottom. Suspension allows greater freedom of movement, balance, lift, and stabilization. Limb devices provide buoyancy to the arms or legs. This type of equipment includes items that attach to the upper arms or ankles, hand-held items, and free-floating equipment that can provide support to the entire body and/or the limbs. Hand-held and free-floating buoyancy equipment are especially effective for strength training (pushing and pulling the equipment through water) and assisting with stretching (e.g., the equipment is placed under the leg to provide more buoyancy during a hamstring stretch). Some of the more popular buoyancy equipment includes:

- Flotation Belts
- Buoyancy Cuffs
- Noodles/Horses
- Buoyant Dumbbells/Barbells
- Kickboards
- Foam Shoes/Platforms
- Water Logs

Never use any piece of buoyancy equipment as a life-saving device.

Surface Area Equipment

Surface area equipment increases the size of the surface area of the body part working in the water. It does not increase the buoyancy properties of a moving object. As explained in Chapter 2, increasing the surface area of an object moving through water creates greater drag, which increases movement resistance and exercise intensity. Equipment of smaller size or with a flat surface is easier to move through water than pieces that are larger or have an irregular surface. While surface area equipment can provide increased overload to enhance strength training in the water, these types of devices should not be used at the expense of proper body alignment and form during activity. Examples of the most common surface area equipment include:

- Paddles
- Non-buoyant Dumbbells

- Webbed Gloves/Aquatic Mitts
- Training Fins
- Ankle/Wrist Fins
- Resistance Buoys/Bells
- Resistance Boots
- Aquatic Parachutes

Land/Water Integration Equipment

Some land exercise equipment can be effectively used in the aquatic environment with little or no alteration. Using land/water integration equipment provides land exercisers an opportunity to transition into water with familiarity. More importantly, aquatic participants can perform slightly modified land exercises in water using land equipment to make the transition from water to land seem less daunting.

Using land equipment in aquatic exercise creates a unique opportunity to use the properties of water to their full advantage. For example, an aquatic exercise "step" (designed for water use only) can provide an excellent opportunity to develop balance skills. Examples of land/water integration equipment include:

- Aquatic Steps
- Tethering Devices
- Resistance Bands/Tubes
- Balls (air-filled, weighted, or foam)

It is important to ensure that participants are using devices appropriate for their individual fitness level, skills, and abilities. Aquatic fitness professionals are responsible for becoming familiar with the different types of aquatic exercise equipment, their purpose (including water properties involved in their use), and the skill level required for proper use.

Progression With Equipment

With land-based exercise, repetitive-training activity at the same intensity level may yield initial results, but eventually participants will plateau. Progression is needed to keep participants interested and moving toward their fitness goals. Their bodies must be continually exposed to increasing levels of intensity to achieve fitness gains. For example, an 8-pound biceps curl using free weights on land may be very challenging for a beginner. But, if performed regularly, this same amount of weight will provide only a minimal challenge in mere weeks, and larger weights will be needed to increase strength gains in the biceps.

Exercise in the water environment is no different, and participants must continually progress movement intensities to achieve fitness gains. One of the benefits to the many types of aquatic equipment is that each challenges participants in a different way. Participants who are exposed to a multitude of devices experience a cross-training effect, because different pieces require unique balance and stabilization skills for proper exercise performance. Before selecting equipment for a certain class, consider the goals for each component of that session. Are participants hoping to improve their cardiovascular fitness, flexibility, muscular strength and endurance, or functional activities of daily living (ADLs)? It is your responsibility as an instructor to become well-acquainted with the different categories of equipment described in this chapter and their roles in intensity progression, and to accommodate as many skill levels as possible within each class. For example, gloves and belts are generally low-intensity equipment choices, while steps and fins are usually near the high end of intensity progression.

Some facilities only have access to a limited variety of aquatic exercise devices and, therefore, participants will repeatedly use the same piece of equipment without access to a "more intense" type. For detailed information on progression, see Chapter 5.

Chapter Five

Teaching Aquatic Exercise

One of the biggest mistakes made by aquatic exercise instructors is poor class design, which results from inappropriately using the medium of water as a teaching tool. To teach aquatic exercise well, you must do much more than just put on a bathing suit, get in the pool, and lead a "low-impact class" at a slower pace. Simply teaching land-based exercises in the water environment will benefit neither the exercisers nor the instructor, because the class will be ineffective. Several key factors differentiate water classes from land-based group fitness, and a full understanding of these is required to teach effectively.

Teaching Methods

The pool can be one of the most challenging environments for a fitness instructor, because often poor acoustics and pool design limit the ability to be seen and heard by participants. Therefore, it is critical to choose the appropriate teaching method for each environment to provide the safest, most effective, and fun water workout. Basically, you have three options when teaching: on the deck, in the water, or a combination of both. For each method, there are advantages and disadvantages, and the best method may vary from pool to pool, or class to class.

The Aquatic Exercise Association (2000) recommends deck instruction as the most effective and safe from the participant's perspective, although it is admittedly the most challenging. Another teaching option, presented by Mary Sanders and Debbie Miles-Dutton, is to have participants either watch the instructor demonstrate a new exercise in the water or watch a video of the new move (YMCA of the USA, 2000). With these techniques, participants have a visual image in mind when the movement is cued, and it provides them an opportunity to ask questions to ensure proper understanding of the move.

Teaching From the Deck

Advantages

- All participants can be observed for safety, to better provide feedback and to pace the workout to individual fitness levels.
- Verbal cues can be given with less voice stress.
- Visual cues can be provided and responded to quickly.
- Participants can more easily observe body position and alignment.

Disadvantages

- Demonstrating impact options can be challenging without proper training on the technique to execute movements on deck.
- Instructors must watch for overheating due to both heat and humidity on land.
- The deck is a hard surface on which to exercise, and can become slippery when wet.

Teaching Tips

- Always wear shoes with traction that will protect from impact.
- Keep movements low-impact, and use a training mat to minimize impact.
- Teach suspended moves from a chair or stool.
- Be careful that the land demonstration of water movements is at the appropriate pace as should be performed by participants in water.
- Instruct through cues and demonstrations, but don't perform all movements throughout class on land.
- Instruct from different positions around the pool to protect the necks of the participants in the front row from hyperextension.
- Dress professionally and comfortably.
- Wear sunscreen, sunglasses, and protective clothing if outdoors.

Adapted with permission from Aquatic Exercise Association, 2000 & Sanders, 1999, 3, WaterFit/Wave Aerobics: www.waterfit.com.

Teaching In the Water

Advantages

- The instructor experiences the same workout environment, feeling work the same way the participants do.

- Participants can receive hands-on corrective feedback and assistance.

- Having the instructor work "with" them motivates some participants.

- It is safer and can be more fun for the instructor.

Disadvantages

- It is difficult for participants to see exactly what a movement should look like.

- It can be more difficult for participants to hear cues and quickly understand an exercise description.

- It is harder for you to see all the participants in class to assess their self-pacing, form, and enjoyment.

Teaching Tips

- Wear shoes with good water traction.

- Keep verbal cues clear and concise.

- Visual cueing signals need to be high above the water so all participants can see and understand them.

- Circulate through the pool during class to provide individualized feedback.

- Use waterproof cue cards to illustrate basic moves.

- Ask for participant feedback on where they are feeling the effects of certain moves, to check for proper execution.

Adapted with permission from Aquatic Exercise Association, 2000 & Sanders, 1999, 3, WaterFit/Wave Aerobics: www.waterfit.com.

The Combination Teaching Method

Advantages

- Participants have a visual image and can see and hear clearly, while also getting hands-on feedback and motivation when you are in the water.

- Safety and pacing are accomplished from the deck, while you can also experience the same workout environment as the participants when in the water.

Disadvantages

- It can be very challenging transitioning from pool to deck and back.

- The deck can become even more wet and slippery.

- It can be confusing for newer participants who don't understand the transitions.

Teaching Tips

- Safe entrances and exits must be used during transitions, with the lifeguard especially alert when your back is turned.

- Provide clear cues to keep moving before transitions are made.

- Take time after transitions, as needed, to readjust to gravity or buoyancy.

- Pre-plan which moves will be taught from the deck, and ask

  participants continually throughout class if they have any questions.

- Wear clothing that will be comfortable both in and out of the water with minimal adjustments.

Adapted with permission from Aquatic Exercise Association, 2000 & Sanders, 1999, 3, WaterFit/Wave Aerobics: www.waterfit.com.

Verbal Introduction

Every class should begin by introducing yourself and describing the class format. Announcements should be made before class begins, in clear concise language, with the music off. While making the announcements, instruct participants to perform large muscle movements to get warm (such as jogging). Identify any new participants and question them about possible health concerns (pregnancy, arthritis, etc.).

Water depth must be explained, especially to new participants to guide them to the appropriate level. And all participants should be encouraged to remain in their selected water depth as much as possible throughout class. Identify participants less confident in their swimming skills or intimidated by the aquatic environment, and urge them to select a working position in which they will feel most secure, such as near a wall or the pool steps. Point out all pool entrances, along with steps and slope changes. Review basic water-safety skills (e.g., recovery to standing), and explain any equipment that will be used. Point out in the beginning of class, as well as throughout the workout, that participants are responsible for pacing their workouts to meet their individual needs. While completing the verbal introduction, observe participants and make any necessary changes to their location in the pool, such as water depth and visibility/distance. All of this is essential to responsibly teaching aquatic exercise, and to minimize risk and maximize enjoyment and effectiveness.

Water Depth

The water depth participants choose will affect their body alignment, movement control, and impact level. Three working water depths can be used in an aquatic exercise class (Figure 16). When training in *shallow* water, the appropriate depth is between navel- and heart-height. In shallow water classes, the feet are firmly planted on the pool bottom, and the body weightbearing percentage is reduced from 50% (waist-level depth) to almost 85% (heart-level depth). Shallow-water training is best suited for participants with greater body fat, which provides more buoyancy and allows them to float more. Non-swimmers who may be uncomfortable at deeper water levels might also prefer shallow water, as may athletes training for power so they can maximize weightbearing activity while minimizing injury potential (e.g., vertical jump training, walking/running). Most shallow-water exercise is performed at heart level.

Transitional water depth is defined as between heart- and neck/shoulder-level. As in shallow water, the feet touch the pool bottom. However, because the lungs are submerged and buoyancy is greater (gravity is reduced by 85% to 90%), support of the feet by the pool bottom is less stable. Transitional water depth can be used most effectively by combining and modifying shallow- and deep-water movements. Additionally, buoyancy belts can help participants to maximize resistance, making their workout more effective.

Deep-water exercise is performed at heart-to-neck depth (90% gravity reduced), with the lungs completely submerged and the feet off the pool bottom. Because the center of buoyancy (which is at the lungs when submerged) is farther

Figure 16a
Shallow water
depth

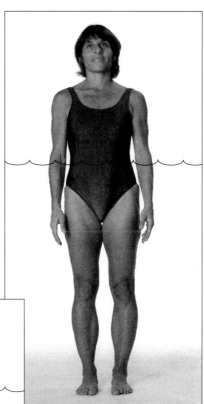

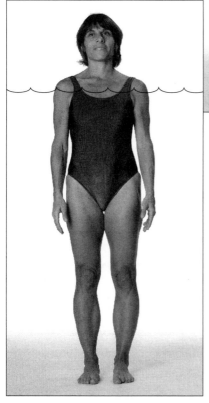

Figures 16b
Transitional
water depth

from the center of mass (the pelvic girdle), finding balance and stability can be very challenging. Although the feet may be able to touch the pool bottom in deep water, they provide minimal support due to the effects of buoyancy. If the exerciser is using buoyancy equipment to be fully suspended in the deep water, the feet are not a support base. Regardless of whether or not the feet are in contact with the pool bottom, exercises performed in deep water do not involve contact with the ground, requiring participants to work while suspended in the water.

It is important to note the distinction between shallow- and deep-water exercise. Differences exist not only in the water depths at which movements are performed, but also in movement selection, design, and implementation. It is best to instruct shallow-water exercise classes first, as these are more like land-based exercise with which you may be more familiar. Proper instruction of deep-water classes requires additional education and training, many of which are not covered in this text.

One vital consideration over which you have little control is pool depth and slope. Shallow-water exercise is most easily performed by most people in water of 3 to 4½ feet, with a slight slope in the pool bottom to accommodate exercisers of varying heights. Because of a sloping pool bottom, participants should face several directions during class, to minimize any imbalances that might occur. Shallow-water exercise is not a good idea in pools with a severely sloped bottom for safety reasons (possible slipping, body misalignment, uneven footing). Deep-water exercise is usually performed at water levels of 6 feet or deeper, and pool slope is inconsequential because exercises are performed in the suspended position.

Pool Temperature and Thermoregulation

Water temperature and thermoregulation can have the greatest impact on aquatic exercisers' comfort, which can impact their enjoyment and long-term participation in aquatic fitness. When designing aquatic exercise programs, it is important to understand that heat loss occurs more rapidly in water than in air. A variety of factors affect heat loss in water, including body-fat levels (body fat slows heat loss in water) and water temperature. The amount of heat lost depends on the temperature gradient between the body and the pool water (Powers & Howley, 1994).

According to the Aquatic Exercise Association (2000), water temperatures between 83° and 86° F (27° and 30° C) allow the body to work normally to achieve fitness benefits, without worry of overheating or heat conservation. Intensity level, however, is a factor in determining the ideal water temperature. The YMCA of the USA (2000) agrees that most healthy adults are comfortable exercising at moderate intensity at the temperatures specified above. Depending on the population and class design, however, specific recommendations exist for water temperature (Table 5.1).

Table 5.1
Water Temperature Recommendations

Population	°F	°C
Competitive athletic training	80–83	27–28
Fitness classes	84	29
Functional water fitness classes	84–86	29–30
Arthritis classes	83–88	28–31
Aquatic therapy	88–90	31–32

Advise participants of the importance of thermoregulation, maintaining core body temperature with a balance of heat production and heat loss. Although you may have little control over pool temperature, it should affect class design. For example, if water is colder one morning, the class should be more active with few if any movement pauses, to maintain body temperature. Usually, the challenge is to avoid cooling rather than worry about overheating. Ideally, design a program that allows participants to keep warm and comfortable throughout the entire class. Techniques to accomplish this include combining upper- and lower-body movements simultaneously, and alternating work with smaller muscle groups with vigorous work using large muscles. Clothing designed to minimize heat loss can also help participants limit body cooling. Examples of such items include chill vests, therapy suits, or tights.

Injury Prevention

Preventing injury should be foremost in your mind at all times. Present correctional cues for injury prevention as a part of the verbal introduction of each class, as well as interspersed throughout class. The first injury prevention method is to select the appropriate water depth for each individual's fitness and skill levels. The main factor in establishing water depth is the individual's body composition and overall comfort and control of movement. Instruction on self-pacing is equally important, and modifications for all intermediate or advanced movements should be provided for participants who are less capable or fit. Provide encouragement and feedback to participants regarding modifications. Implementing and enforcing all pool safety standards is key to injury prevention.

Proper movement execution is another key factor in preventing injury during aquatic exercise classes. Regularly teach proper movement patterns for even the simplest exercises (e.g., walking or jogging). Participants should be instructed and encouraged to maintain neutral spinal alignment and correct body mechanics during all movements. Common errors that can cause injury include locked knees, a rounded or hunched back, hyperextension of joints at the wrist, shoulder, neck, or spine, and excessive plantar flexion (performing exercises entirely on the toes with contracted calves) (Figures 17–19). Demonstrate movements clearly and correctly, and provide modifications as needed.

Water shoes can be used to provide traction and avoid slipping during class and while entering/exiting the pool. Also, balance can be problematic for many water exercisers, and they therefore need options to help maintain balance (e.g., sculling, grounded versus suspended, or holding onto the pool wall). Lastly, aquatic exercise participants need to be cued regularly on breathing, as well as monitoring and adjusting intensity to meet their personal fitness and skill levels.

Because of the properties of water, there are few "contraindicated" movements in aquatic exercise. There are, however, certain moves that are higher risk than others that should usually be avoided, especially by certain populations. For the purposes of this publication, "high risk" is defined as any movement that has a significantly greater potential risk of injury for most participants. More clearly stated, it is any

Figure 17
Neck positions are extremely important to watch for, especially if you are teaching from the deck while participants are in the water.
a. Hyperextended neck
b. Neutral neck

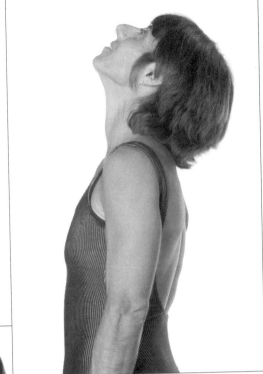

a.

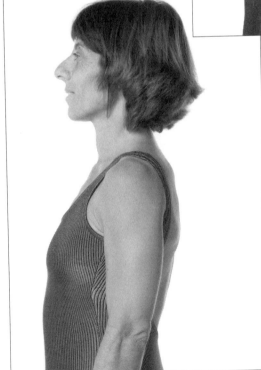

b.

Figure 18

A rounded back is improper working form and should be avoided.

a. Excessively rounded upper/mid back

b. Proper neutral spinal alignment

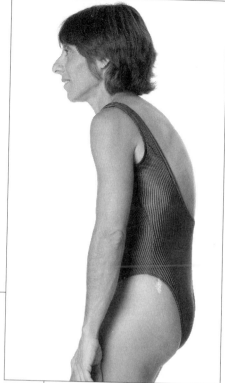

a.

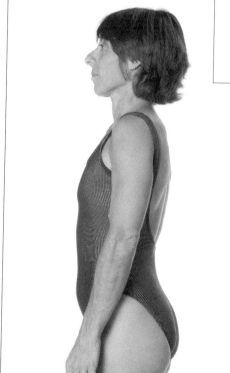

b.

Figure 19
Locked knees should be
avoided for all exercises
in water, just as on land.
a. Locked knee
b. "Soft" knee

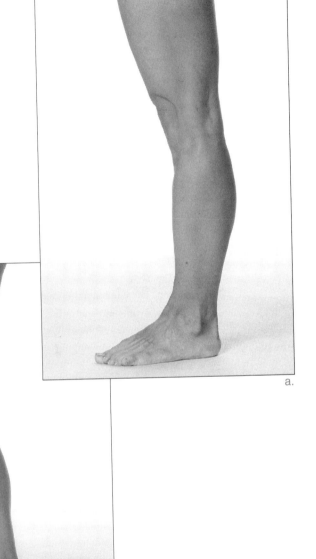

a.

b.

movement that most participants are unable to perform with proper form. It is your responsibility to evaluate every exercise for its safety, effectiveness, and suitability for each class and each participant. If a higher-risk movement is included in the class design, demonstrate alternatives to minimize risk of injury. Examples of higher-risk movements in the water are presented in Table 5.2.

Table 5.2
High-risk Water Movements

- Very-high-impact exercises (e.g., high jumping in extremely shallow water)

- Very fast movements (e.g., moves performed at land pace), including fast movements that transition from above the surface to below, which can cause joint stress

- Extended use of the arms overhead, which causes injury through shoulder fatigue, and improper body alignment that leads to back pain

- Moves that create/increase muscle imbalances or poor body alignment

- Prone flutter kicks that cause back hyperextension if the body is not appropriately braced

- Wall hanging exercises that stress the shoulders, arms, wrists, or fingers

- Hip flexion versus abdominal conditioning, as it is ineffective and potentially harmful to the back by creating/adding to muscle imbalances

- Knee hyperflexion during quadriceps stretches

- Knee hyperextension during hamstring stretches

- Any moves that compromise spinal integrity (e.g., full neck circles, moves that arch a portion of the back excessively)

Pool Safety

An important part of responsibly teaching aquatic exercise involves understanding and complying with pool safety standards. Shirley Archer, J.D., M.A. (1998), has compiled a checklist of items for instructor safety, which is presented in Table 5.3. This checklist includes preventive measures you should take to protect both yourself and water participants.

Table 5.3
Water Fitness Instructor Safety Checklist

Take the following preventive measures to protect yourself and participants:

- Take basic water safety training geared for non-lifeguards, such as the YMCA Aquatic Safety Assistant course or the American Red Cross Basic Water Rescue program.

- Maintain certification in standard first aid and CPR.

- Review the pool's emergency action plan, introduce yourself to the lifeguards, and understand how to communicate with rescue staff in an emergency.

- Know the location of the rescue equipment and first aid station.

- Do not simultaneously serve as a lifeguard and an instructor.

- Understand proper incident reporting.

- If your clientele includes non-swimmers, know who they are and be able to teach recovery to a stand and how to float in water.

- Learn how to spot signs of panic, active drowning, and passive drowning. Unless you are a trained and certified lifeguard, do not attempt to rescue a drowning person yourself; instead, notify the lifeguards.

- Since panic often contributes to drowning, encourage people who do not know how to swim to enroll in basic swimming lessons.

- Prior to the class, check the decks and pool access for any hazards. Also make sure you can easily see the pool bottom and are aware of any "drop-offs" to deeper levels.

- Immediately report any hazards you may notice. If a hazard cannot be removed and will interfere with the safety of class participants, do not conduct your class.

- Foster open communication with participants to encourage feedback.

- Inform participants of the importance of proper footwear; it provides support, protects the soles of the feet, and prevents slipping.

- If participants need to wear corrective vision glasses in the pool to see you, encourage them to do so.

- If outdoors, have participants face away from the sun so they can see you, and advise them to wear sunscreen, hats or visors, and sunglasses.

- Know the policies and procedures for outdoor and indoor pool closure due to inclement weather.

- Encourage participants to wear appropriate exercise attire, drink plenty of water, maintain good postural alignment, and work at their own pace.

- Wear good footwear to provide support and prevent slipping.

- On deck, use safe demonstration techniques to minimize impact.

- Develop good visual cueing skills to spare your voice.

- If outdoors, drink plenty of water and protect yourself with sunscreen, sunglasses, and a hat or visor.

- Understand how to use electrical outlets, stay informed about electrical safety issues, and be aware of the danger of electrical shock. Electrical outlets should not be closer than 10 feet to the pool.

Archer, 1998. Reproduced with permission of IDEA, The Health & Fitness Association, (800) 999-IDEA or (858) 535-8979: www.ideafit.com.

Participant supervision is one of the most critical concerns of aquatic exercise instruction. Be familiar with the warning signs of distress in the water, such as flailing arms and cries for help. Adequate lifeguard supervision for the number of participants in the pool is gravely important. No "universal rules" govern the ratio of required lifeguards to pool users, because requirements vary by pool and according to local city/county guidelines. However, it is important that you not be solely responsible for the safety of aquatic exercisers during class. You cannot perform the functions of both instructor and lifeguard under any circumstances, and must not be afraid to cancel a class should this situation arise (Archer, 1998).

> Be sure that qualified, alert, adult lifeguards are stationed in elevated positions above the pool during a water exercise class. Under absolutely no circumstances should you simultaneously perform the duties of both lifeguard and instructor, regardless of your training or experience.

Hydration

A widespread misconception on the part of aquatic exercise participants is that they don't sweat during water exercise, and therefore hydration is not as critical in water as it is when exercising on land. This, of course, could not be further from the truth. Sweat loss in water occurs just as rapidly as it does on land. It is just not noticeable, because in the pool sweat is carried away from the body by the water, which is different from the evaporative cooling that occurs in air. Encourage participants to drink fluids before, during, and after their water workouts, and remind them to drink before they're thirsty because the thirst mechanism is not sufficient to ensure adequate hydration.

Heart-rate Monitoring

The tried-and-true method for determining exercise intensity on land is through heart-rate monitoring. Because of the direct relationship between exercise intensity, oxygen consumption, and heart rate, this method is both accurate and sufficient. In water, however, the heart-rate response to exercise can be up to 13% or 17 beats per minute lower than during comparable land exercise (Maybeck, 2000). Research has demonstrated that hand-held equipment use during aquatic exercise increases heart rate with little cardiorespiratory benefit. Further, it has been shown that cool water reduces heart rates while warm water yields higher heart rates, and that exercise in shallow water versus deeper water elicits higher heart rates comparable to land exercise versus deeper water (YMCA of the USA, 2000).

The reason exercise heart rate is lower in deeper water has not yet been clearly defined. There are currently several viable theories, all of which use sound reasoning and any of which may be accurate. The temperature theory proposes lower heart rates in deeper water are due to the cooling effect of water on the body. Because cooling occurs with less effort in water than in air, the heart has to work less to meet the demands of the body, and heart rate is lower. The gravity theory is based on the reduced effect of gravity on the body when submerged. Venous return of blood to the heart from the lower body requires less effort, which in turn reduces exercise heart rate. The compression theory involves the effects of water's hydrostatic pressure on the body. When submerged, water acts as something of a compressor on the vascular system that reduces the venous load to the heart (similar to the gravity theory). Lastly, the partial pressure theory proposes that the more efficient gas exchange of oxygen in the blood reduces the heart's workload. It is thought that oxygen (a gas) enters the blood (a liquid) more readily when under the pressure of the water, as described by the physics law of partial pressure.

Whatever the reason, because of lower heart rates during deep-water exercise, heart-rate monitoring alone is not the preferred method for determining exercise intensity. Aquatic fitness experts agree that the best way to get an accurate measure of exercise intensity in water is to combine the rating of perceived exertion (RPE) and talk test (breathing rate) methods. Heart rates should be used as an adjunct to these two methods, and their meaning interpreted with a water heart rate chart. If a special condition requires the precise monitoring of heart rate, a heart rate monitor should be used. Monitors provide a more accurate ongoing measurement than a brief pulse count. Pulse counts usually require a decrease or cessation of movement to measure, which slows the heart rate almost instantly in water (more abruptly than on land) and provides an inaccurate assessment of workload.

Intensity Progression

Participants in aquatic exercise classes should be encouraged to work at an intensity level of "somewhat hard" to "strong" on the RPE scale, similar to the guidelines recommended for land-based fitness. It is critical that they also pace themselves and regulate their own intensity so they are appropriately challenged without overexerting themselves. Participants can alter the intensity of their workouts by changing the speed at which they work or the size of their movements. If a particular movement is too intense or complicated, suggest an easier movement to substitute in its place.

The *Speedo Aquatic Fitness Instructor's Training Manual* (Sanders & Rippee, 1993) defines intensity progression as "a method of increasing or decreasing the workload by varying a component of the move to gradually change the degree or level of physical demand." To progress participants through a cardio-vascular conditioning movement, first have participants perform the most basic version of the move. Progression is accomplished by increasing the movement size, force, and speed, or adding to the lower-body load. This last variation occurs by moving to shallower water, adjusting the working position to rebounding, or adding surface area equipment to the lower body if suspended in deep water. During a muscle conditioning exercise, progression occurs by increasing the effort and speed, traveling, and adding overload equipment (Sanders, 1999, 1). Table 5.4 presents tips for teaching movement progression to participants, after ensuring that they are aware of the exercise objective.

Table 5.4
Tips for Teaching Movement Progression

Teaching progression tips are listed below. Always be sure that participants have done a thorough thermal warm-up and know the workout objectives.

Teach   Teach the basic move.

Instruct proper alignment and neutral posture.

Teach the functional objective of the exercise.

Coach   Cue the primary movers, and practice the movement pattern.

Adjust the size of the move, monitoring range of motion.

Cue correct posture and biomechanics.

Cue proper breathing.

Progress resistance overload, adding force, increasing speed, or traveling.

Respond Observe and respond to the class.

Remind participants to regulate personal intensity by adjusting movement size and/or speed.

Check body mechanics.

Encourage and celebrate good performance.

Provide feedback that is personal, positive, and specific.

Monitor intensity (RPE, Talk Test).

Encourage self-pacing.

Take a water break.

Reduce intensity and begin a new progression.

Adapted from Sanders & Maloney-Hills, 1998. Reprinted with permission, *ACSM Health and Fitness Journal.*

Chapter Six

Programming

nstructors need many of the same skills to teach aquatic
exercise classes that are needed to teach land-based group
exercise classes. However, land instructors are often
challenged when learning to teach aquatic fitness. Not only
is the use of water principles in program design a challenge, but
the effects of water on movement speed can be troublesome for
new instructors when designing and demonstrating aquatic
exercise moves for participants of variable fitness, skill, and
ability levels.

Class Format

Traditional water fitness classes include the following
segments:

- Thermal warm-up (3–10 minutes)
- *Optional* pre-stretch (3–5 minutes)
- Cardiorespiratory warm-up (3–5 minutes)
- Cardiorespiratory training (20–60 minutes)
- Cardiorespiratory cool-down (3–5 minutes)
- Muscle conditioning work (5–15 minutes)
- Post-stretch (5–10 minutes)

All aquatic classes should begin with a thermal warm-up,
which serves a similar purpose to the warm-up in a land-based
class, to increase core temperature, lubricate the joints, and
stimulate delivery of oxygen to working muscles. The pre-stretch
is an optional component that can be added; however, most
aquatic fitness professionals and class formats currently extend
the rhythmical warm-up and eliminate the pre-stretch (Aquatic
Exercise Association, 2000). The brief static stretches in the pre-
stretch should not be performed unless water temperature is
adequate to maintain body warmth while stretches are being
held. If temperatures are not as warm as desired, the pre-stretch
can be completed by keeping the body moving as much as
possible while stretching (for example, keeping the arms moving
while performing a calf stretch). Unlike the thermal warm-up,
the cardiorespiratory warm-up is designed to begin overloading
the cardiovascular and respiratory systems in preparation for
the more vigorous movements to come. Because the respiratory
and heart rates begin to increase in the thermal warm-up, many
instructors choose to blend the thermal warm-up, pre-stretch,
and cardiorespiratory warm-up into one continuous segment.

Either way is appropriate, as long as the goals of the warm-up segments are met.

Movement Suggestions for Warm-up

- Beginning at a low intensity, and gradually progressing to a moderate intensity

- Sculling and jogging in shallow or deep water

- Jogging with breaststroke in shallow water, arms slicing

- Pushing and pulling while kicking in shallow or deep water

- Pushing down in shallow or deep water

- Performing scissor and jumping jack moves in shallow or deep water

Active Warm-up of Major Muscles

- Quadriceps: kick front, progress to neutral kick front, pressing arms back

- Hamstrings: jog with heels coming up behind

- Tibialis anterior/ankles: ankle circles

- Pectorals: breaststroke with the arms thumbs up

- Rhomboids/trapezius/latissimus dorsi: reverse breaststroke

- Abductors/Adductors: easy jacks; wide jog

- Gluteals: hug one knee toward the chest and hop on the supporting leg

- Low back: pelvic tilt with hands on hips

Adapted from Sanders, 1999, 3, with permission from WaterFit/Wave Aerobics: www.waterfit.com.

The cardiorespiratory portion of an aquatic fitness class can run anywhere from 20 to 60 minutes, as prescribed in the American College of Sports Medicine guidelines for cardiorespiratory training (ACSM, 1998). The goal of the cardiorespiratory training segment of an aquatic fitness class is to maintain an elevated heart rate while performing continuous rhythmic activity (the same as in land-based classes). Closely monitor intensity, and continually remind participants to pace themselves. Aerobic intensity should gradually increase to a peak and then gradually decrease, leading into the cardiorespiratory cool-down. The cool-down allows the respiratory and heart rates to decrease slowly in preparation for the slower-paced muscle-conditioning segment of class.

The purpose of the muscle-conditioning segment is to develop muscle strength and/or muscle endurance by exercising specific muscle groups. With careful design and the use of aquatic equipment (although equipment is not necessary), some instructors integrate the muscle strength and endurance work into the aerobic portion of class. If equipment is used for muscle conditioning, the exercises chosen must be specific to that equipment and appropriate for the level of the class.

The aquatic exercise class should end with some type of final stretch segment, to develop range of motion and flexibility and reduce the likelihood of muscle soreness. While static stretches are the best way to develop flexibility, water temperature may prohibit the holding of stretches long enough to maximize flexibility benefits.

Take care to maintain participants' core temperature while stretching. Warmth can be preserved by keeping the rest of the body moving while each muscle group is stretched, or by mixing mild thermal warm-up movements between stretches. The overall goal is to provide participants with a stretch segment that allows them to leave the pool feeling both warm and relaxed.

Alternative Class Formats

A variety of class format options are available to the aquatic fitness instructor. While it is beyond the scope of this book to provide detailed explanations of these many options, a few possibilities are briefly described. Additional class formats not described here include classes that focus only on resistance or flexibility training, deep-water fitness classes, water walking/jogging classes, and even newly developed formats like water tai chi. Classes for special populations are discussed in a later section of this chapter.

Circuit Training

Circuit-training classes allow participants to circuit through stations of specific activities. Station segments usually alternate between three to five minutes of aerobic training and one to two minutes of muscular conditioning, and may or may not involve the use of equipment (Aquatic Exercise Association, 2000). Some circuits are designed with stations focused specifically on balance, agility, flexibility, plyometric training, muscular strength, and muscular endurance. The circuit-training class format works well with men, athletes, and self-motivated participants. The benefit to circuit training is that is it interactive, informal, and fun. Because they are challenging to instruct, circuit classes can be taught to the group as a whole, or may be self-guided.

Interval Training

While circuit training involves both aerobic and resistance training, interval training focuses exclusively on aerobic conditioning. Interval formats alternate bouts of high-intensity aerobic (or possibly anaerobic) work with recovery bouts of low-intensity, passive aerobic work. Work intervals at higher intensity can last anywhere from 30 seconds to three minutes, based on the abilities/level of the class. And cycles are patterned in a ratio of high intensity to low intensity from 1:3 to 3:1 (Aquatic Exercise Association, 2000). While previously thought to be best-suited for athletes seeking sports-training work or well-conditioned exercisers at low risk of injury, interval-training techniques are now known to be a safe and effective way to maximize training effects for just about any population.

Aquatic Step Training

Step training, one of the most popular land-based classes, can be performed in water with an aquatic bench. Step exercise in water can safely provide benefits for both cardiorespiratory and muscular endurance, as long as the appropriate water depth is chosen, the pool slope is not too excessive, and movements are properly designed (Aquatic Exercise Association, 2000). Step training in water decreases impact stress, while increasing work against gravity (Sanders & Rippee, 1993). Plyometric movements, such as hopping and jumping, using the step in water are effective to train the lower-body musculature and improve cardiorespiratory performance (Evans, 1996). Further, step training in water can help older adults train for activities of daily living (Sanders & Kennedy, 1998). It should be noted, however, that simply leading a land-based step class in water is not appropriate, and does not yield fitness benefits (Evans, 1996). Research has demonstrated that movements in any water class, whether utilizing the step or not, should be paced at one-third to one-half the speed of comparable land movements. Speed should only be increased when faster movements can be performed with proper body mechanics (Sanders & Kennedy, 1998).

Tips for Instructing Aquatic Step Training

- Make sure participants have mastered basic water skills without the step before participating in an aquatic step workout.

- Help participants find the appropriate water depth for stepping, probably deeper than normal to protect from impact but not so deep that the overload effects of gravity are minimized.

- Participants should be able to maintain proper body alignment, should not have to lean forward, and should be able to work their hands through the water and move with control at all times.

- Practice sculling for balance/coordination and recovery from falling while stepping, as these stabilization skills will feel different from atop a step.

- Working positions should be reviewed away from the step.

- To minimize movement of the step during class, have participants center their weight and foot placement on the step, and be sure to allow enough movement time for balance and to use the water's resistance.

- Progress intensity and complexity slowly (enlarging moves, coordinating upper- and lower-body movements), reminding participants constantly to select the intensity level that is right for them regardless of any other participants.

Personal Limitations

nstruct participants to follow their own health and fitness limitations when selecting movements and pacing themselves during a class. It is your responsibility, however, to be aware of the possible personal limitations of the participants, and to design and implement movements accordingly. Fatigue can be a significant problem for participants lacking the muscular strength and endurance required to move continuously in water for an entire class. Learn to recognize the signs of fatigue and instruct participants in ways to decrease movement intensity.

Age is also a consideration. Older adults may need softer music, louder cues, aid with equipment selection, and different choreography options than younger or more athletic participants. Other personal limitations include health conditions and exercise goals. Some older adults, for example, seek health-related fitness benefits, rather than cardiorespiratory or strength conditioning. And, some special populations are drawn to the water to improve their ability to perform ADLs, and movement options will need to accommodate their differing goals and abilities. One other personal limitation may be participant height, as participants who have longer arms and legs will need more time to execute movement patterns and transitions than shorter participants.

Special Populations

Working with special populations is both challenging and rewarding, and it is also inevitable in the water environment. Water's supportive environment makes it an ideal exercise medium for people with all types of health concerns, both chronic and acute. Aquatic classes will often include participants with conditions such as hypertension, diabetes, obesity, heart disease, or arthritis. People with disabilities or recovering from injury are also drawn to aquatic exercise classes. Exercise can improve all of these participants' health and quality of life, and aid them in managing their condition. Considering this, you need to be well-versed in the types of special populations that will likely show up in your classes. You will also need to know how to provide modifications for these populations, and be clear on your role in working with these participants.

First and foremost, any person requiring special modifications due to a medical or physical condition of any kind must obtain a physician release before beginning an exercise program. In most cases you are merely responsible for verifying that individuals have been cleared for activity in the water. However, more detailed procedures may exist at some facilities. Know when to refer participants to a more qualified medical professional. If a participant has a condition with which you are unfamiliar and/or unprepared to deal, it is imperative they be referred to appropriate medical personnel. Keep in mind at all times that your scope of practice is limited to general, fitness-specific health care. What follows is brief information on some of the most commonly seen special populations in aquatic exercise, and pertinent guidelines for working with these participants in an aquatic fitness class.

Pre-/Post-Natal

With the comforting properties of buoyancy and hydrostatic pressure, it is not surprising that aquatic fitness is popular among women during pregnancy and postpartum. Buoyancy counteracts gravity to reduce weightbearing and joint stress, while hydrostatic pressure increases stroke volume, and plasma and blood volume, which reduces exercise heart rate and lower-leg swelling associated with pregnancy (Campion, 1990). Pregnant and postpartum exercisers often experience physio-logical changes, including increased blood volume, decreased oxygen availability, musculoskeletal changes, and emotional changes, all of which require you to take special consideration when planning and teaching (ACOG, 1994). While normal procedures for dealing with special populations must be followed for pre-/post-natal exercisers, additional programming issues need to be addressed. Table 6.1 provides a list of tips for working with pre-/post-natal women when teaching an aquatic fitness class. These tips need to be implemented in classes designed specifically for pre-/post-natal participants, as well as for any pre-/post-natal participants who may be "mainstreaming" themselves into a non-specialized water fitness class.

Table 6.1
Tips for Working with the Pre-/Post-Natal Water Exerciser

- The warm-up should be longer by up to 10 minutes, to allow for adjustments to buoyancy and the unique cardiac demands of pregnancy.

- The cardiovascular component of class should be slightly shorter because of the limited availability of oxygen during pregnancy.

- The strengthening portion of class should target the abdominals, spinal extensors, quadriceps, gluteals, and the upper body.

- Kegel exercises for the pelvic floor should be included in every class.

- The flexibility section of class should include an unloaded cool-down to promote relaxation, and be sure to stretch the pectoral and cervical muscles.

- Emphasize proper body mechanics at all times to prevent injury and prepare participants for the physical demands of motherhood (lifting a baby, pushing a stroller).

- Intensity should be monitored using the "talk test" and RPE method (12–14 on the 6–20 Borg scale).

- Be sure to cue proper breathing and avoidance of the Valsalva maneuver.

- For more information on pre-/post-natal exercise, contact the American College of Obstetricians and Gynecologists (ACOG) at (202) 863-2518.

Adapted from Norton, 1998. Reproduced with permission of IDEA, The Health & Fitness Association, (800) 999-IDEA or (858) 535-8979: www.ideafit.com.

Older Adults

Older adults (age 55+) are the fastest growing segment of the population. Older adults also make up the greatest number of persons with chronic conditions, and are historically most likely to participate in aquatic exercise programs (YMCA of the USA, 2000). Aquatic fitness provides older adults with an excellent way to enhance quality of life by providing training benefits for functional abilities and fitness level, as well as providing an enjoyable social experience. Older adults do, however, have a wide array of special needs and limitations, and you need to be prepared to meet those needs with extra attention, modifications, and patience. Table 6.2 presents exercise considerations for working with older adults in the aquatic environment.

Table 6.2
Tips for Working with the Older Adult Aquatic Exerciser

- Lengthen the warm-up to allow more time for increased circulation, joint warmth, and elevation of core temperature.

- Teach and progress all movements gradually, allowing time for repetition to aid in learning each movement pattern.

- Encourage socialization and group interaction to facilitate friendships and potentially alleviate loneliness or depression.

- Be aware of the greater need to be seen and heard, as many older adults have hearing or vision troubles; also watch music volume!

- As much as possible, provide individualized care, instructing with one-on-one feedback to teach basic skills and modifications.

- Be sure to present the objectives of an exercise and relate its value in terms the older adult will value, such as lifting grandchildren or carrying groceries.

- Research the effects of common medications on exercise (e.g., anti-hypertensives, beta-blockers, diuretics).

- Instruct and interact at all times with patience and care.

Arthritis

With the number of Americans with arthritis estimated at more than 40 million (Nieman, 2000), be prepared for arthritic individuals in the pool environment. Although exercise was previously thought to worsen the chronic condition of arthritis, it is now known to benefit people with osteoarthritis and a host of rheumatic conditions, including rheumatoid arthritis, fibromyalgia, and gout. In fact, current evidence points to the likelihood that a significant portion of disability found in arthritic individuals is caused by a lack of fitness (Nieman, 2000). When exercise programs are correctly designed within their abilities, people with arthritis can safely improve their health and fitness, gaining both strength and aerobic fitness with no detrimental effects on affected joints (Ettinger, 1998; Van Baar, Assendelft, & Dekker, 1999; Van den Ende et al., 1998).

The term arthritis actually refers to more than one hundred different diseases that involve swelling, pain, and limited joint and connective tissue movement throughout the body (Arthritis Foundation, 1999). A chronic condition that usually lasts a lifetime, it currently has no known causes or cures. Symptoms come and go, alternating between flare-ups and remission. Urge participants with arthritis to minimize activity when symptoms flare up, as movement is both painful and difficult. Arthritis research has shown that disease sufferers have less joint range of motion, decreased aerobic capacity, and weaker muscles than people of the same age without arthritis (Nieman, 2000). Special training, such as that offered by the Arthritis Foundation, is required to become qualified to instruct an aquatic exercise class for people with arthritis. Table 6.3 lists general information on working with arthritics in a non-specialized aquatic fitness class,

keeping in mind that people with arthritis need to be cleared for
physical activity.

Table 6.3
Tips for Working with Arthritic Participants in Water

- If changing is difficult, encourage participants to wear swimwear to the pool under their clothing.

- Guide participants in selecting appropriate water depth, noting that weightbearing decreases as water depth increases.

- Ballistic, higher impact moves should be avoided.

- Movements should occur from a neutral joint position at all times, and be stopped if they cause pain. Look for and correct participants with locked or stiffened joints.

- Encourage participants to exercise at their own pace, and not overexert themselves or perform more repetitions than comfortable.

- Coach participants to breath in a normal rhythmic pattern, and slow down if they find themselves "running out of breath."

- Progress movements gradually and perform them slowly, so participants move their joints to the point where a gentle stretch is felt.

- Breaks need to be offered frequently so muscles can rest between exercises.

- Never assist any participants in moving body parts.

- If joints are painful, red, hot, or swollen exercise should be discouraged.
  NOTE: In all cases, each participant should follow his or her physician's guidelines.

- Movements that are painful or restricted should be executed with a limited range of motion and decreased surface area, and at slower speeds.

Adapted from Sanders & Maloney-Hills, 1999 with permission from WaterFit/Wave Aerobics: www.waterfit.com.

Post-rehabilitation

The healing properties of buoyancy, adjustable resistance, and
compression (hydrostatic pressure) make aquatic exercise one of
the most effective ways to rehabilitate an injured body part in
preparation for the return to land activity. Physical therapists

have long used water therapy to facilitate recovery from injury, and you need to understand your role when dealing with post-rehab participants. Aquatic classes should be used to help recovering participants strengthen their injured area, while maintaining fitness and overall function as much as possible (Larue, 1997). All post-rehab participants need to be cleared for activity. Keep in mind that your role is NOT that of physician, chiropractor, or physical therapist, but of a fitness professional helping participants make the transition from rehab to land with the use of water training. Table 6.4 presents program design considerations for working with post-rehab clients in the aquatic fitness setting.

Table 6.4
Post-rehab Water Training Tips

- For muscle strains or tendinitis, avoid resisted exercise for the involved area if painful, keep intensity minimal by moving slowly without overload equipment, and strengthen opposing muscle groups using water's buoyancy.

- For low-back pain, teach participants to work at all times with a neutral spine (working with their back against the pool wall if necessary). Limit the range of lower-extremity moves such as hip extension, use hand moves for balance and use a buoyancy belt in shallow water to assist balance and decrease compression. Perform moves only in a straight plane (no rotation) and only allow participants to progress to deeper water if all movements can be executed with a neutral spine.

- For general post-surgical participants, avoid rotary movements and perform range of motion moves in straight planes. Avoid ballistic and rebound moves of the involved joint. Keep moves at limited range of motion at first, and decrease the size and speed of the movements as needed.

- For knee conditions, avoid rotary, quick, snapping knee movements and complicated choreography. Work at decreased speeds with smaller moves, and only stretch to the end of the pain-free range of motion in warm water. Progressions should be gradual for squat moves or aquatic stepping.

Adapted from Hill & Sanders,1997. Reproduced with permission of IDEA, The Health & Fitness Association, (800) 999-IDEA or (858) 535-8979: www.ideafit.com.

Music

S electing appropriate music is a challenge faced by all fitness instructors. Regardless of the exercise modality or class type, the important aspects of music selection are motivation, suitability, style, and enjoyment by both the instructor and the participants. Consider both your preferences and your participants', and choose music that will create enthusiasm and fun for everyone. One key way to ensuring a motivating and effective class for all participants is to provide a variety of music to accommodate the different age groups and tastes of participants. Select music styles that are familiar to the participants in class. For example, when teaching a group of mostly older adults, hard rock or rap music is probably not appropriate; styles like swing and big band music, however, will probably be very well received.

In an aquatic exercise class, the warm-up music should be stimulating and make the participants want to move through the water. As the class progresses to the cardiovascular component, motivation can come from music with a strong steady beat, even though participants are not necessarily moving in time to that beat. During muscle endurance and strength work, where explanations and correctional cues occur more frequently, background music is the preferred choice (perhaps classical or instrumental). This type of music encourages participants to work at their own pace during the exercises rather than trying to keep up with the beat of the music. During the stretching and flexibility segment of the class, the music should be somewhat less vigorous and intense, although water temperature is a factor. If the temperature permits, slow, relaxing music can be used while static stretches are held. If the water is cooler, a less calming music selection is called for to encourage movement while stretching (YMCA of the USA, 2000).

Music level is another vital concern. Depending on pool acoustics and accessibility to a microphone, the pool environment may not be conducive to loud music. Additionally, aquatic classes often include seniors who may have hearing difficulties. Loud music will serve only to drown out your voice, making instruction more difficult to hear and the class less enjoyable for participants. To avoid this, regularly ask participants if they can hear the cues. Encourage them to ask you to turn down the volume if it becomes too loud at any time during class.

Music tempo is another key concern for aquatic fitness professionals. The beat of the music in aquatic fitness classes is used for motivational purposes rather than actual movement timing, as it is often not as possible to "move to the beat" in water as it is on land. The Aquatic Exercise Association (2000) recommends a music tempo of 125–150 beats per minute for shallow-water exercise, using one-half- or one-quarter-time per movement repetition. The cadence is dependent on the age and skill level of class participants, as well as any resistance equipment being used. Therefore, successful aquatic programs may utilize music at either a slower or faster pace than this recommendation. Irrespective of water depth, participants are the overall deciding factor in selecting music tempo for any aquatic fitness class. They should be able to perform all exercises with a full range of motion and complete control while maintaining proper body alignment (Aquatic Exercise Association, 2000; Gardiner, 1996).

Index

A

abdominal crunch with
noodle, 32
acceleration, 18
action/reaction, 10, 14–15, 22
active drowning, 62
activities of
daily living (ADLs), 8, 74
adductor stretch, 35
adhesion, 15
aerobic fitness, 8–9
age, 76, 79
agonist/antagonist
muscle balance, 16
alternative class formats, 73–75
American College of
Obstetricians and
Gynecologists, 78
American College of Sports
Medicine, 4–5, 71
American Red Cross Basic
Water Rescue program, 62
anchored position.
See extended position
ankle/wrist fins, 43
aquatic exercise
and aerobic fitness, 8–9
athletic training, 8–9
benefits of, 2–4
and bone loss prevention, 7
and cardiorespiratory fitness,
4–5
and flexibility, 5–6
functional training, 8
growth of, 2
versus muscle land work, 13
and muscular conditioning, 5

teaching, 46–47
therapeutic benefits, 7–8
and weight management, 6
Aquatic Exercise Association, 2,
47, 55, 84
aquatic exercise equipment, 14,
28, 38–39, 72
buoyancy equipment, 28,
41–42
criteria for selecting, 39–41
land/water integration, 40,
43–44
progression with, 44–45
surface area equipment, 42–43
water-specific, 40
aquatic fitness instructors,
skills and knowledge, 10
*Aquatic Fitness Professional
Manual*, 13
aquatic mitts, 43
aquatic moves
basic cardiovascular moves,
24–27
basic muscle-conditioning
moves, 27–37
aquatic parachutes, 43
aquatic step, 43, 74
aquatic step training, 43, 74–75
aquatic stretches, 33–37
Archer, Shirley, 62
arm movements, 26
arthritis, 80–81
Arthritis Foundation, 80
athletic stance, 22
athletic training, 8–9

frog-leg jumps, 27
functional training, 8

G

gastrocnemius stretch, 33
gloves, webbed, 28, 30, 43
gout, 80
gravity theory, of lower
    heart rate in deep water, 65

H

hamstring stretch, 34
hand-held buoyancy
    equipment, 41
health conditions, 76
heart-rate monitoring, 65–66
height, 76
high-risk moves, 57, 61
hip-flexor stretch, 36
Hoeger, W., 5
hopping, 74
horses, 42
hydration, 64–65
hydrostatic pressure, 4, 8,
    10, 17, 65–66, 77
hyperextended neck, 58
hypertension, and water
    depth, 17

I

IDEA Fitness Programs Survey, 2
incident reporting, 62
inertia, 10, 16–17, 18
injury prevention, 2–3, 56, 57
intensity
    and action/reaction principle,
        14–15
    and drag forces, 13–14
    and inertia, 16–17
    of jumps, 27

monitoring, 72
    progression, 66–67
    and water temperature, 55
interval training, 73–74

J

jogging, 25
joint motion, 8
jumping, 26–27, 74
jumping jacks, 27
jumping with a twist, 27

K

Kegel exercises, 78
Kennedy, Carol, 4
kickboards, 31, 42
kicking, 25–26

L

land/water integration
    equipment, 43–44
leaps, 27
leverage, 10, 19
levers, 19, 26
lifeguards, 62, 64
limb equipment, 41
locked knees, 57, 60
loud music, 79, 84
lunge, 31

M

mambos, 25
medical referral, 77
medications, effect of on
    exercise, 79
mid-trapezius/rhomboid
    stretch, 34
Miles-Dutton, Debbie, 22, 47
mitts, aquatic, 43

modifications, 56
muscle-conditioning moves,
    5, 27–37, 72
muscle land work versus
    water exercise, 13
musculoskeletal injury, and
    vertical alignment, 12
music, 83–84
music tempo, 84
music volume, 79, 84

N

neutral neck, 58
neutral position, 23–24
neutral spinal alignment,
    57, 59, 82
Newton, Isaac
    First Law of Motion
        (Law of Inertia), 16
    Third Law of Motion, 14
non-swimmers, 62
noodles, 32, 42

O

older adults, 76, 79

P

paddles, 42
panic, 62
partial pressure theory, of lower
    heart rate in deep water, 65–66
passive drowning, 62
pectoral stretch, 37
pendulum, 26
personal limitations, 75–76
physical therapists, 81
physician release, 77
plantar flexion, 57
plyometric training, 9, 74

pool depth, 52–54, 56
pool safety, 62–64
pool slope, 54
post-rehabilitation
    exercisers, 81–82
post-stretch, 72
postural stability, 4
pre-/post-natal exercisers,
    77–78
pre-stretch, 70
programming, 69
    alternative class formats,
    73–75
    class format, 70–72
personal limitations, 75–76
special populations, 76–82
progression, 3
    with aquatic exercise
        equipment, 44–45
    aquatic step training, 75
    cardiovascular conditioning, 67
    muscle conditioning, 67
    tips for teaching, 68
pulse count, 66

Q

quadricep stretch, 36

R

rating of perceived exertion, 66
ready position, 22
rebound position, 23
recovery to standing, 21
rehabilitation, 7–8
rescue equipment, 62
resistance, 10, 15–16, 18, 19, 27
resistance bands/tubes, 43
resistance boots, 43
resistance buoys/bells, 43
rheumatoid arthritis, 80

rocking, 26
rocking horse, 26
rotary movements, 82
rounded back, 57, 59
running, 25
Russian kicks, 26

S

safety, 51, 62–64
Sanders, Mary E., 24, 47
Sanford Center on Aging,
    University of Nevada, Reno, 8
scissors, 27
sculling, 21–22, 75
self-pacing, 56
shallow water exercise, 52, 53, 54
shoes, 48, 49, 57, 63
shoulder adduction with
    dumbbells, 29
soft knees, 60
special populations, 76–77
    arthritis, 80–81
    older adults, 79
    post-rehabilitation, 81–82
    pre-/post-natal, 77–78
speed, 10, 17, 18, 74
Speedo Aquatic Fitness
    Instructor's Training
    Manual, 67
squat with kickboard, 31
stabilization skills, 20, 21–22, 75
static stretches, 70, 72
step training, aquatic, 43, 74–75
straight plane, 82
stretching, 33–37, 70, 72
surface area, 10, 19
surface area equipment, 42–43
suspended position, 24

T

tai chi, water, 73

talk test, 66
teaching aquatic exercise,
    46–47
    combination method, 50
    from the deck, 47, 48
teaching methods, 47–50
    verbal introduction, 51
    in the water, 49
temperature, 55, 70
temperature theory, of lower
    heart rate in deep water, 65
tethering devices, 43
therapy suits, 56
thermal warm-up, 70, 71
thermoregulation, 55, 56
tights, 56
training fins, 43
transitional water exercise, 52, 53
traveling, 27–28
traveling jumps, 27
tricep extension with webbed
    gloves, 30
Tsukahara, N., 7

V

Valsalva maneuver, 78
verbal introduction, 51, 56
vertical alignment, and
    musculoskeletal injury, 12
video instruction, 47
viscosity, 15, 16
visual cueing skills, 63
$\dot{V}O_2$, 5

W

walking, 25
water depth, 52–54, 56
water heart rate chart, 66
water logs, 42
water-resistance equipment, 14
water-safety skills, 51

water-specific aquatic exercise
    equipment, 40
water temperature, 55, 70
webbed gloves, 28, 30, 43
weight management, 6
weightbearing conditions, in
water, 11–12
whole-body buoyancy
    equipment, 41
Wilbur, R. K., 8
working positions, 23–24

Y

YMCA, 55
YMCA Aquatic Safety
    Assistant course, 62

References & Suggested Reading

Abraham, A., Szczerba, J.E., & Jackson, M.L. (1994). The effects of an eleven-week aqua aerobic program on relatively inactive college age women. *Medicine & Science in Sports & Exercise*, 26, 5, S103.

American College of Obstetricians and Gynecologists. (1994). Exercise during pregnancy and the postpartum period. Washington, D.C.: American College of Obstetricians and Gynecologists.

American College of Sports Medicine. (1997). *ACSM's Exercise Management for Persons with Chronic Diseases and Disabilities.* Champaign, Ill.: Human Kinetics, Inc.

American College of Sports Medicine. (1998). Position Stand: The recommended quantity and quality of exercise for developing and maintaining cardiorespiratory and muscular fitness, and flexibility in healthy adults. *Medicine & Science in Sports & Exercise*, 30, 6, 975–991.

American Council on Exercise. (1993). *Aerobics Instructor Manual.* San Diego, Cal.: American Council on Exercise, 296–302.

American Council on Exercise. (1998). *Older Adult Manual.* San Diego, Cal.: American Council on Exercise.

Aquatic Exercise Association. (1999). *The AEA Water Well.* Nokomis, Fla.: Aquatic Exercise Association, 6.

Aquatic Exercise Association. (2000). *Aquatic Fitness Professional Manual*, 2nd ed. Nokomis, Fla.: Aquatic Exercise Association.

Archer, S.J. (1998). Water exercise liability. *IDEA Health and Fitness Source*, February, 71–77.

Arthritis Foundation. (1999). Arthritis Fact Sheet, available at www.arthritis.org

Arthritis Foundation & National Council of the YMCA of the USA. (1996). *Arthritis Foundation YMCA Aquatic Program*. Atlanta: The Arthritis Foundation.

Baretta, R. (1993). Physiological training adaptations to a 14 week deep water exercise program. Unpublished dissertation, University of New Mexico, Albuquerque.

Becker, B. & Cole, A.J. (1997). *Comprehensive Aquatic Therapy*. Boston, Mass.: Butterworth-Heinemann.

Bravo, G., Gauthier, P., Roy, P.M., Payette, H., & Gaulin, P. (1997). A weight-bearing, water-based exercise program for osteopenic women: Its impact on bone, functional fitness, and well-being. *Archives of Physical Medicine and Rehabilitation*, 78, 12, 1375–1380.

Bushman, B.A., Flynn, M.G., Andres, F.F., Lambert, C.P., Taylor, M.S., & Braun, W.A. (1997). Effect of four weeks of deep water run training on running performance. *Medicine & Science in Sports & Exercise*, 29, 5, 694–699.

Campbell, K.D., et al. (1990). Effect of water exercise on body composition in overweight females. *American Alliance for Health, Physical Education, Recreation and Dance*, Annual Convention Presentation, New Orleans, LA.

Cassady, S.L. & Nielsen, D.H. (1992). Cardiorespiratory responses of healthy subjects to calisthenics performed on land versus in water. *Physical Therapy*, 72, 7, 532–538.

Coven, E. & Sidelman, S. (1996). Dealing with medical emergencies in seniors' classes. *IDEA Today*, October, 71–77.

Curry, M. (1997). Water Fitness 101. *IDEA Today Fitness Handout: Taking the Plunge into Water Fitness*, June.

Diamond, B. (1997). Training water fitness instructors. *IDEA Today*, April, 25–29.

Erner, H.K., & Hoeger, D. (1995). Is water aerobics aerobic? *Fitness Management*, 11, 5, 29–30.

Ettinger, W.H. (1998). Physical activity, arthritis, and disability in older people. *Clinical Geriatric Medicine*, 14, 3, 633–640.

Evans, E. (1996). Can water exercise tip the scale? *IDEA Today*, May, 27–30.

Forster, R.F. (1997). Water Healing. IDEA, Water Fitness Conference Presentation, Anaheim, Cal.

Gardiner, J. (1996). Choosing music for seniors. *IDEA Today*, January, 66–67.

Gwinup, G. (1987). Weight loss without dietary restriction: Efficacy of different forms of aerobic exercise. *American Journal of Sports Medicine*, 15, 3, 275–279.

Herbert, D.L. (1999). Emergency response plans must be in writing. *Fitness Management*, 15, 7, 24–26.

Hills, C. & Sanders, M.E. (1997). Water fitness teaching guidelines for postrehabilitation. *IDEA Today*, October, 75.

Hoeger, W., et al. (1993). A comparison of selected training responses to water aerobics and low-impact aerobic dance. *National Aquatics Journal*, 13, 6.

IDEA. (1999). Client Handout: Ready to dive into water fitness? *IDEA Health and Fitness Source*, May, 80.

Kennedy, C. & Sanders, M.E. (1995). Strength Training Gets Wet! *IDEA Today*, May 24 – 30.

Kolovou, T. & Eksten, F. (1998). Water sports training. IDEA Health & Fitness Source, June, 50–58.

Koury, J. (1996). Aquatic Therapy Programming Guidelines for Orthopedic Rehabilitation. Champaign, Ill.: Human Kinetics Publishers, Inc.

Landgridge, J. & Phillips, D. (1988). Group hydrotherapy exercises for chronic back pain sufferers. Physiotherapy, 74, 269–273.

Larue, L. (1997). Postrehabilitation Water Fitness. *IDEA Today*, October, 71–74.

Maybeck, J. (2000). Aqua Beat – Heart Rate Monitors Make a Splash! *The AKWA Letter*, 13, 6, 9 & 13.

Miles-Dutton, D. (1996). Water fitness for beginners. *IDEA Today*, September, 29–30.

Nieman, D.C. (2000). Exercise soothes arthritis. *ACSM'S Health & Fitness Journal*, 4, 3, 20–27.

Norton, C.O. (1998). Pre/postnatal water exercise. *IDEA Health & Fitness Source*, April, 55–59.

Powers, S.K. & Howley, E.T. (1994). *Exercise Physiology* (2nd ed.). Dubuque, Iowa: Brown & Benchmark, 245–258.

Ruoti, R.G., Troup, J.T., & Berger, R.A. (1994). The effects of nonswimming water exercises on older adults. *Journal of Orthopaedic and Sports Physical Therapy*, 21, 6, 655–661.

Ryan, P. (2000). Fitness programs trend report. *IDEA Health & Fitness Source*, January, 53–55.

Sanders, M., Constantino, N., & Rippee, N. (1997). A comparison of results of functional water training on field and laboratory measures in older women. *Medicine & Science in Sports & Exercise*, 29, ixx.

Sanders, M.E. (1999, 1). Cross over to the water. *IDEA Health & Fitness Source*, March, 53–58.

Sanders, M.E. (1999, 2). Water fitness for older adults. *IDEA Health & Fitness Source*, December, 23–28.

Sanders, M.E. (1999, 3). *Specificity of Training and Deep Water Program.* WaterFit/Wave Aerobics, www.waterfit.com.

Sanders, M.E. (2000). Land training + water training = best results. *ACSM'S Health and Fitness Journal*, 4, 2, 34–36.

Sanders, M.E. & Kennedy, C. (1998). Water research update. *IDEA Health & Fitness Source*, June, 33–39.

Sanders, M.E. & Maloney-Hills, C. (1998). Aquatic exercise for better living on land. *ACSM'S Health & Fitness Journal*, 2, 3, 16–23.

Sanders, M.E. & Maloney-Hills, C. (1999). *The Golden Waves Program, Functional Water Training for Health.* WaterFit/Wave Aerobics, www.waterfit.com.

Sanders, M.E. & Rippee, N.E. (1993). *Aquatic Fitness Instructor's Training Manual.* London, U.K.: Speedo International Limited.

Simmons, V. & Hansen, P. (1996). Effectiveness of water exercise on postural mobility in the well elderly: An experimental study on balance enhancement. *Journal of Gerontology*, 51A, M233–M238.

Smit, T. & Harrison, R. (1991). Hydrotherapy and chronic lower back pain: A pilot study. *Australian Journal of Physiotherapy*, 37, 229–234.

Sova, R. (1992). Water Walking. *The AKWA Letter*, 6, 4.

Stemm, D. (1993). Effects of aquatic simulated and dry land plyometrics on vertical jump height. Unpublished master's thesis, Philadelphia, Penn.: Temple University.

Suomi, R. & Lindaur, S. (1997). Effectiveness of arthritis foundation program on strength and range of motion in women with arthritis. *Journal of Aging and Physical Activity*, 5, 341–351.

Templeton, M.S., Booth, D.L., & Kelly, W.D.O. (1996). Effects of aquatic therapy on joint flexibility and functional ability in subjects with rheumatic disease. *Journal of Orthopaedic and Sports Physical Therapy*, 23, 376–381.

Tsukahara, N., et al. (1994). Cross-sectional and longitudinal studies on the effect of water exercise in controlling bone loss in Japanese post-menopausal women. *Journal of Nutrition and Science Vitaminology*, 40, 1, 37–47.

Twynham, J. (1998). Wading through the sea of water equipment. *IDEA Health & Fitness Source*, June, 43–49.

Van Barr, M.E., Assendelft, W.J., Dekker, J., et al. (1999). Effectiveness of exercise therapy in patients with osteoarthritis of the hip or knee: A systematic review of clinical trails. *Arthritis and Rheumatology*, 42, 7, 1361–1369.

Van den Ende, C.H., Vlieland, T.P.V., Munneke, M., et al. (1998). Dynamic exercise therapy in rheumatoid arthritis: A systematic review. *British Journal of Rheumatology*, 37, 6, 677–687.

Wilber, R.K., Moffatt, R.J., Scott, B.E., Lee, D.T., & Cucuzzo , N.A. (1996). Influence of water run training on the maintenance of aerobic performance. *Medicine & Science in Sports & Exercise*, 28, 8, 1056–1062.

YMCA of the USA, Sanders, M.E. (ed). (1999). *Teaching Swimming Fundamentals*. Champaign, Ill.: Human Kinetics Publishers, Inc., 80–88, 109–115.

YMCA of the USA. (2000). *YMCA Water Fitness for Health*. Champaign, Ill.: Human Kinetics Publishers, Inc.

NOTES

NOTES

NOTES

NOTES

NOTES

NOTES

ABOUT THE AUTHOR

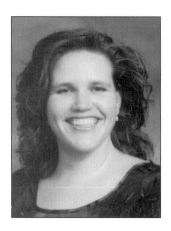

Sabra Bonelli, M.S., is the head of the Fitness Programs
Department for the Mission Valley YMCA in San Diego, Calif.
Bonelli received her master's degree in exercise physiology
from San Diego State University. She has authored several
ACE Fit Facts and articles in *ACE Certified News,* as well as ACE's
Step Training specialty book. Bonelli is a member of ACE's
Group Fitness Instructor Examination Committee.

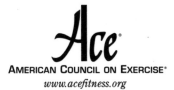

AMERICAN COUNCIL ON EXERCISE®

www.acefitness.org

YES, I would like to receive information on the following ACE certifications:

- ❏ Lifestyle & Weight Management Consultant
- ❏ Group Fitness Instructor
- ❏ Personal Trainer
- ❏ Clinical Exercise Specialist

Name _____

Address _____

City_____ State_____ ZIP_____

Home Phone (_____)_____

Work Phone (_____)_____

E-mail _____

AMERICAN COUNCIL ON EXERCISE®

www.acefitness.org

YES, I would like to receive information on the following ACE certifications:

- ❏ Lifestyle & Weight Management Consultant
- ❏ Group Fitness Instructor
- ❏ Personal Trainer
- ❏ Clinical Exercise Specialist

Name _____

Address _____

City_____ State_____ ZIP_____

Home Phone (_____)_____

Work Phone (_____)_____

E-mail _____

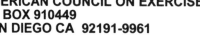

BUSINESS REPLY MAIL

FIRST-CLASS MAIL   PERMIT NO. 22113   SAN DIEGO, CA

POSTAGE WILL BE PAID BY ADDRESSEE

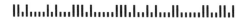

**AMERICAN COUNCIL ON EXERCISE
PO BOX 910449
SAN DIEGO CA 92191-9961**

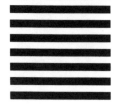

BUSINESS REPLY MAIL

FIRST-CLASS MAIL   PERMIT NO. 22113   SAN DIEGO, CA

POSTAGE WILL BE PAID BY ADDRESSEE

**AMERICAN COUNCIL ON EXERCISE
PO BOX 910449
SAN DIEGO CA 92191-9961**